ASMR
for Beginners

by Julie Young and Ilse Blansert (TheWaterwhispers)

GARRICK
STREET
PRESS

Publisher Mike Sanders
Associate Publisher Billy Fields
Executive Acquisitions Editor Lori Hand
Cover/Book Designer William Thomas
Development Editor Kayla Dugger
Production Editor Jana M. Stefanciosa
Indexer Tonya Heard
Layout Ayanna Lacey
Proofreader Monica Stone

First published in 2015 in the United States by DK Publishing
6081 E. 82nd Street, Indianapolis, Indiana 46250

001–316091–JAN2019

This 2019 edition is published by Garrick Street Press, an imprint of
Dorling Kindersley Limited

ISBN: 978-1-4654-8885-5
Library of Congress Catalog Number: 2018967851

*To Connie: a dear friend whose inspiration placed me on the path to writing this book.
I am forever grateful. —Julie
To my grandmother, who gave me one of my first real-life ASMR experiences and
who introduced me to Bob Ross. —Ilse*

Contents

Appendixes

Introduction

Autonomous sensory meridian response, or ASMR, is a tingly feeling that begins in the head or scalp, is caused by recognizable sounds that you hear every day, and results in a deep feeling of relaxation. Popularized on YouTube by folks known as *ASMRtists* who make videos to stimulate the tingly sensation and promoted by ASMR experiencers, what was once an online subculture has gone mainstream and is causing the clinical community to sit up and take notice. While some question its scientific validity, others swear by it, saying it is a safe and natural, with no harmful side effects.

Though we come from two very different backgrounds, we both know how hard it can be to turn off the noise of the day and relax. As longtime ASMR experiencers, we've both turned to the internet in search of the sounds and experiences that gave us the tingly feeling that always helped us instantly unwind and relax, and now we are ready to share everything we know about the ASMR experience with you.

You don't have to be a physician, a researcher, or even an ASMR experiencer to learn more about this fascinating phenomenon. Many people who come to the world of ASMR do so because they have heard about it from someone else, or they stumbled upon it accidentally. If you are already a "tingle head," this book will help you gain a deeper understanding about the sensation you are already familiar with and where it comes from. It will also help you understand what is truly happening inside the brain when that ASMR feeling occurs.

Let us take you on a journey inside the mind to learn what the ASMR phenomenon is and how you can use it to relax or get a good night's sleep at last!

How This Book Is Organized

This book is divided into five parts:

Part 1, ASMR Basics, takes you on a journey into the online subculture that has earned national headlines and the interest of some members of the medical community. You learn what ASMR is, what it feels like, and who is affected. We also discuss why it is being called the solution to insomnia and how it has an effect on the stress response.

Part 2, The Origins of ASMR, shows you that even though ASMR is a relatively new idea, it is connected to concepts and practices that are far older. We track the evolution of ASMR and the ASMR community while exploring its history in other well-known and clinically acknowledged practices.

Part 3, Finding Your Triggers, enables you to delve into the sounds that soothe you to discover whether it is possible for you to experience ASMR yourself. You learn why certain vocals, sounds, and well-known scenarios seem to have an effect on people and how you can identify these in your own life.

Part 4, Applying ASMR, starts with ways you can use ASMR techniques with others in everyday life. We then go behind the scenes of ASMR content creation to show you how to write, film, direct, star in, and edit your own ASMR content.

Part 5, Becoming Part of the ASMR Community, begins with some tips for how to be a good ASMR community member, as well as how to deal with others who aren't. We then show you what it takes to build your ASMRtist platform. From networking with others, to social media, to how much you can really expect to make, we cover it all as you join the big leagues.

Extras

Throughout this book, you'll find some handy bits of information in sidebars that give you more information about ASMR.

DEFINITION

Throughout this book, you will find a number of terms that are important to the scientific and ASMR communities. We identify and define these terms in relationship to ASMR in these sidebars while providing you with a listing of these terms in Appendix A.

DID YOU KNOW?

These fast facts apply to the scientific community, as well as the ASMR community, and can be found in the chapters to which they correspond.

TINGLE TIP

These directives are designed to help you get the most out of the topic we cover in each chapter. This may apply to sleep, meditation, hypnosis, or other ASMR-related activities.

KEEP IN MIND

These alert you to any special considerations you'll want to be aware as you learn more about the ASMR phenomenon and its methodologies.

Note: ASMR is not a medical practice, nor should it be used as a replacement for any treatment program prescribed by your physician. Before turning to ASMR as a sleep aid, consult with your health-care professional about whether or not this content may be an option for you.

Acknowledgments

First and foremost, I want to thank Lori Cates Hand for believing in this project when it was still an idea in my head. Thanks also to Ilse Blansert for trusting in a complete stranger to bring the world of ASMR to life and lending her name and expertise to the project. I couldn't have done it without you! I also want to give a big thank you to Dr. Craig Richard at Shenandoah University in Virginia for his enthusiasm and support and for double-checking my science. I think we both learned a lot! And finally, to my friends "Heather Feather," "Whisper Sweetie," and every other ASMRtist who contributed in one way or another to this project, thank you from the bottom of my heart and thank you for being there when my head is humming with outside noise and I need the tingles to take me away. —Julie Young

Thank you everyone at Alpha Books for giving me this incredible opportunity to bring ASMR to a wider audience. Thank you so much to my father, John, who told me that being different and making a difference isn't a bad thing, and his parents, who were the first people to give me tingles. Thank you to my aunt and other grandmother who support my work and spread the word about ASMR whenever they can. Thank you also to my fiancé, Chris, for his love and tech support. Thanks as well to Maria "GentleWhispering," Lilium, and all of my friends in the ASMR community. Last but not least, I want to thank the viewers; without you, I would not be where I am today. Your support keeps me going and I am truly grateful for each and every one of you. —Ilse Blansert

Trademarks

All terms mentioned in this book that are known to be or are suspected of being trademarks or service marks have been appropriately capitalized. Alpha Books and Penguin Random House LLC cannot attest to the accuracy of this information. Use of a term in this book should not be regarded as affecting the validity of any trademark or service mark.

ASMR Basics

It's the pleasant feeling of relaxation that no one can fully explain. Autonomous sensory meridian response (ASMR) is a tingly brain reaction to specific, external stimuli that is being used to help countless people get to sleep at night.

Never heard of it? You're not alone. In fact, many people who have experienced ASMR throughout their lives are surprised to learn that the sensation has a name and that others feel it as well. They are also surprised to learn that there is a thriving online ASMR community; ASMR content creators have turned their webcams into tingle transmitters for their fans, who rely on their videos for natural and effective rest and relaxation.

In this part, we take you on a journey into the internet's new sleep aid that is causing the clinical community and the media to sit up and take notice. We learn how this combination of sound and imagery can trigger the senses to help you de-stress and get a good night's sleep once and for all!

Hooked on a Feeling

Did you ever have a teacher or a friend whose voice was so melodic that just listening to him talk was enough to put you into a trance? Are there certain noises that you find sonically satisfying and that help you relax almost instantly? Have you ever watched fish swim in an aquarium only to become so mesmerized by the monotonous movement and gentle sounds of the filter that your eyes grew heavy and you longed to take a nap? Does the mention of certain activities such as hair brushing, light massage, or a manicure cause your brain to get a warm, fuzzy feeling?

If you answered "yes" to any of those questions, there is a good chance you have experienced ASMR in the past or are capable of experiencing it in the future. It's a question of finding the right content to support your particular triggers.

In this chapter, we take you on a journey inside the mind to learn more about this unique phenomenon that is helping countless people de-stress and get to sleep at night and causing the scientific community to sit up and take notice.

In This Chapter

- ASMR: one tingly sensation
- Is ASMR real?
- The science behind tingling
- How ASMRtists stimulate the senses
- Misophonia: like fingernails on a chalkboard

What Is ASMR?

Autonomous sensory meridian response (ASMR) is a semi-scientific term for a perceptual phenomenon characterized by a pleasurable, tingly sensation that begins in the head and scalp and moves throughout the limbs of the body, causing them to relax. It is an involuntary event that occurs when someone is provoked by visual, auditory, olfactory, and/or cognitive stimuli, such as whispering, tapping, or hair brushing. These provocations, whether they happen in real time or are merely suggested, trigger a subconscious reaction that is very difficult to explain to those who do not experience it.

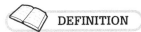

DEFINITION

Autonomous sensory meridian response (ASMR) is a perceptual phenomenon characterized by a tingly feeling in the brain or scalp caused by the experience or suggestion of external stimuli.

ASMR is not new; however, it is new to the mainstream. Thanks to coverage in local, regional, national, and international media, those who have experienced ASMR all of their lives have learned that not only does the sensation have a name, but that others feel it, too, and make up a thriving online community ready to trigger their tingles.

Devon King is typical of those who first experienced ASMR as a child but didn't know what the sensation was or whether anyone else could feel it. After receiving confused looks and head scratches from those he described the strange feeling to, he gave up trying to explain it. He presumed he was endowed with the same special "Spidey senses" that affected his favorite comic book hero. However, unlike Spiderman's superpower, King's tingles did not arise in response to nearby danger. His occurred when he was most at ease and could be caused by a variety of events, such as face painting, watching someone draw or paint, listening to a story, or having his breathing monitored.

Unsure as to whether or not he had a sixth sense or some kind of mental disease, King began to research his condition. However, vague descriptions and imprecise keywords yielded few results. Eventually, he stumbled across an online subculture of people who not only claimed to have experienced the same sensation that he did, but had even given it a name.

The Origins of the Name

Due to the various terminologies used to explain the ASMR experience, it is impossible to know for certain when the subject was first introduced online or whether it has another name that has not been identified. What we do know is that one of the earliest descriptions of the sensation appeared on the Steadyhealth.com message board in 2007. A user created a post in which he asked about "weird head sensations" that occurred intermittently and caused a euphoriclike state within him. The post, which was filed under "nervous system disorders and diseases," prompted a number of responses from those who reported a similar feeling whenever people spoke slowly and carefully or made deliberate gestures with their hands.

Others claimed to be triggered by certain sounds or by watching people complete everyday tasks in a concentrated way. As these people searched for a clinical explanation to the phenomenon, they assigned a variety of names to the condition, including attention-induced head orgasm (AIHO), the weird head sensation (WHS), and the unnamed feeling (UNF). However, in 2010, Jenn Allen of New York coined the term that has been adopted by *tingle heads* everywhere, as well as the community at large: ASMR.

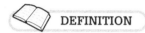

DEFINITION

A **tingle head** is a colloquial name for someone who experiences ASMR.

Although it has not yet been recognized as an official term by the clinical community, some scientists feel it provides a fairly accurate description for the experience it describes:

- **Autonomous:** A behavior that an individual has no control over

- **Sensory:** The type of nerves that transport information to the brain

- **Meridian:** A term from Chinese medical practices; the life energy that flows through the body from its central core

- **Response:** How the body reacts to a specific stimulus or thought

Real or Imagined?

Early on, ASMR skeptics and critics considered the ASMR phenomenon to be nothing short of New Age hokum with a clinical-sounding name. However, today's scientists are less inclined to dismiss it so easily. The sheer number of individuals who have come forward independently and described the same syndrome with uncanny similarity lends credence to its plausibility, even if the condition itself has yet to be conclusively established.

Dr. Steven Novella, an academic clinical neurologist at Yale University School of Medicine and author of the NeuroLogica blog, examined the ASMR phenomenon in March 2012 and concluded that its concept is similar to that of a migraine headache in the fact that they are said to exist based on the fact that so many people have experienced them over the years. However, he was quick to point out that due to the highly subjective nature of the ASMR experience, it is an inherently difficult field to study. Because it is a sensation that can't be seen and is felt and reported by only some, it falls into a scientific blind spot similar to other conditions thought to be myth until someone develops a way to measure them.

While there is much we don't know about ASMR, we do know that there are two types of ASMR episodes that occur among those who experience the sensation:

- **Type A:** These are spontaneous episodes caused by the experiencer without the help of external stimuli. They occur through specific thought patterns, which are unique to the individual. For example, remembering or thinking of something significant and pleasant to you may cause ASMR tingles.

- **Type B:** These are *triggered* by external stimuli and are affected by one or more of the senses, as well as the thought patterns connected to the triggering event. For example, the sound of scissors cutting may be something your brain empathizes with, leading to a tingly sensation.

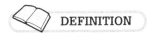 **DEFINITION**

In ASMR terms, a **trigger** is the stimulus that causes the ASMR feeling to occur.

Triggers can vary wildly among those who experience ASMR. We will go into more detail about these triggers in Part 3; however, the most common external triggers include the following:

- Slow, soft, well-enunciated, and/or unique speech patterns

- Educational narrative

- Soothing, empathetic attention from another person

- Music and other pleasurable sounds

- Careful and deliberate task completion

- Hair play, massage, and other touch-based sensations

No matter what the trigger, the result is the same—a silvery, sparkly feeling that creates a euphoric feeling in the body. It is this brain buzz that some believe can help alleviate headaches, relax someone who is stressed, and even put the person to sleep.

But how and why does it work? That is the question that researchers have yet to fully uncover; however, there are a number of emerging theories about how it works, why people experience it, and what areas of the brain are involved. While researchers understand that ASMR includes elements of other clinically proven and often-used stress-management techniques (which will be explored more fully in Part 2), what they can't account for is the goose bump–like feeling that distinguishes an ASMR event from something that is merely relaxing.

Over the years, researchers have suggested that the ASMR sensation may be anything from a small seizure brought on by auditory stimuli to a way of activating the brain's pleasure response. Others speculate that the ASMR phenomenon engages an uncontrollable, primitive area of the brain that reacts to triggers it finds particularly soothing. When the trigger meets with that specific area of the brain, the connections between a person's consciousness and thoughts are separated, which then allows the individual to focus on the sensations he finds innately pleasurable.

Regardless of what is happening in the brain at the time the ASMR feeling occurs, it is possible that some people are simply hardwired to get an extra shot of pleasure from sounds, visuals, and events they find exceptionally satisfying.

TINGLE TIP

ASMR is not the same as goose bumps, although goose bumps may occur during an ASMR experience. Goose bumps are a physiological phenomenon that humans retained from their hairier ancestors, when raising body hairs helped to insulate the body or to make it appear larger when threatened by danger. Humans continue to experience goose bumps in response to different triggers, as well as to the memory of the trigger. The ASMR experience is similar but tends to be more internal in nature and does not always result in raised skin.

Does Everyone Experience ASMR?

Not everyone seems to experience ASMR, although some researchers believe everyone has the potential to experience it, provided they can identify the stimuli that trigger their ASMR experience and recognize the feeling once it occurs.

Generally speaking, the ASMR community is comprised of three groups of people:

- Those whose first ASMR experience occurred in childhood and have had it occur periodically throughout their lives

- Those who thought they were incapable of feeling ASMR but experienced the sensation during their teen years or in adulthood and have continued to do so ever since

- Those who recognize ASMR content as something that is relaxing and soothing but who are incapable of achieving the tingly sensation associated with it

People Who First Experienced ASMR When Young

The people in the first category typically have their first ASMR experience at a young age and often describe a feeling of calm serenity when, for example, their mother played with their hair, a friend lightly tickled the inside of their forearm, or they listened as a teacher carefully and patiently explained the day's lesson. It is a phenomenon that follows them throughout their lives, and when they "discover" the ASMR community, they tend to seek out videos that re-create these real-life experiences.

At least one researcher does not think this early and continued form of experiencing ASMR is a coincidence. Craig Richard, PhD, an associate professor of physiology and cell biology at Shenandoah University in Virginia, an ASMR experiencer, and the founder of the ASMR University blog, suggests the ASMR phenomenon may be something everyone is born with but some are more sensitive to it than others. In July 2014, he published his ASMR Origin Theory in hopes that it would encourage ongoing conversation about the phenomenon, inspire future studies and research, and give theories for further investigation.

Richard believes the physiological response associated with ASMR (the brain tingles) is something that is present at birth and remains with people throughout their lives. He sees a direct connection between the triggers that stimulate the ASMR experience and those that happen naturally through the pathways of interpersonal bonding, whether intentionally or unintentionally.

After studying countless ASMR role-plays online, Richard noticed that all of them contain certain triggers that have been used over the centuries to stimulate and soothe infants and small children, such as the following:

* A raised vocal pitch

* Soft speech and eye contact

* Gentle mannerisms

* Careful movements

He says that regardless of whether the creator of the ASMR video is acting out a medical exam, salon service, or other type of experience, the video contains many of the same elements as those listed previously, and because people are already conditioned to be calmed and nurtured by this kind of stimuli, those triggers continue to work into adulthood, even though they may appear to be entirely different scenarios. Each event being acted out is designed to build trust and to connect individuals to one another.

Richard says that when people experience the ASMR feeling, they may also be releasing endorphin molecules, which can stimulate pleasure relaxation and sedation. These endorphins may also be responsible for the feeling of euphoria associated with the ASMR experience because the brain is receiving information it believes to be safe, trustworthy, and preferable. Endorphins are known to be a powerful stimulant for dopamine release. This, according to Richard, "helps you recall, recognize, and focus on things in your life that trigger endorphins, whether it is a yummy food, the comfort of a parent, your best friend, or a romantic partner."

Endorphins are also known to stimulate oxytocin, another molecule that may be central to the ASMR process. This neurotransmitter and hormone is often called the *love drug*. Oxytocin is most likely responsible for the sense of comfort and relaxation and decreased stress levels that occur during the ASMR event.

DID YOU KNOW?

Oxytocin also stimulates serotonin, which gives individuals a sense of satisfaction and well-being and is also part of the ASMR experience. Dr. Richard notes that most anti-depression medications boost serotonin levels; therefore, the mood-lifting experience reported by some in response to ASMR experiences could be due to the oxytocin-stimulating serotonin production.

People Who First Experience ASMR Later in Life

The second category of ASMR tingle heads are those individuals who come to the sensation a little later in life and whose ASMR episode may have happened by accident. During this kind of event, the individual is suddenly triggered by a combination of sights, sounds, and actions that create an ideal environment for the ASMR experience, even if it's never happened before. Those who fall into this category may include individuals who have recently changed doctors or who interact with hair dressers or other service professionals whose vocal timbre, hand gestures, and environmental noise can set the stage for an ASMR event. When an ASMR episode occurs by surprise, it can be unsettling for someone unaccustomed to it.

At its core, this ASMR category employs the same elements associated with the first category and may be connected to infancy and endorphins, as Dr. Richard suggests. Somehow, though, the connection gets lost for a period of time until the person comes back into contact with something that triggers him later in life.

People Who Do Not Experience ASMR

The final category is made up of those who find the soothing voices and white noise associated with ASMR calming and who may even be able to go to sleep to the content. However, their experience does not include the tingly, sparkly sensation affiliated with the event. It is this category that gives experts pause and causes them to wonder whether some people are simply immune to the ASMR phenomenon or merely have yet to find a trigger that causes the tingles to occur.

Richard speculates the reason some people simply can't experience ASMR is that their body may not produce the appropriate amount and types of molecules and receptors involved in the ASMR sensation. This biological difference may also explain why some infants are harder to soothe than others, or why some people are hypersensitive to sounds, textures, and other stimuli.

"In addition to genetics, these molecules and receptors could be influenced by the environment, diet, disorders, toxins, drugs, and even childhood experiences and cultural norms," he says.

 TINGLE TIP

Not sure what ASMR feels like? Consider purchasing a head-massaging tool that looks like an open-ended egg beater (also known as a *head scratcher*). This tool has been known to create the tingle sensation for those who may never have experienced ASMR and can re-create it for those who have.

Stimulating the Senses

No matter where you fall on the ASMR spectrum, it is an extremely personal event. In order for the ASMR sensation to occur, the individual must make a connection to the sensory stimuli on a neurological and emotional level, even if he has no connection to the creator. (Sometimes this connection also happens in the unconscious mind, so the viewer might not even be aware of the connection while watching or experiencing this even in real life.)

This fluctuates greatly from one person to another and is not a one-size-fits-all proposition. The sounds must hit the right frequency in the brain, visuals must be pleasing to the eye, and the experience must be one that enables the individual to open up and trust. When a viewer is able to trust the ASMR atmosphere, he can surrender to the sensation and let the tingles take him away.

The Role of ASMRtists

In order to help individuals achieve the ASMR sensation, content creators known as *ASMRtists* strive to create the perfect blend of sound, image, and suggestion that will cause viewers to succumb to relaxation or a peaceful slumber. The resulting content ranges from simple sound assortments to full-blown role-plays complete with elaborate scenery and special effects. No matter how intricate or modest the content may be, it tends to fall into one of the following categories (which we will explore more fully in Part 3):

- **Vocal:** These tend to be word heavy and feature whispered/soft dialogue along with slow, deliberate speech patterns, mouth sounds, and enunciation.

- **Art and music:** These can stand alone or complement another experience, but are designed to stimulate individuals on a multisensory level through the audio/visual combination.

- **Nonvocal sound:** Similar to a white noise machine, sound-only content offers an array of auditory stimuli, including scratching, tapping, page turning, water pouring, and more.

- **Visual:** These feature slow, careful hand gestures and soft gazes, and can include educational tutorials, household tasks, and craft construction, among others.

- **Personal attention:** These can come in a variety of forms, but usually include a soothing one-sided conversation in which the ASMRtist offers the viewer plenty of TLC.

- **Tactile:** These typically re-create the sounds and sensations associated with a specific touch or event and may include medical examinations, grooming, light touch, and more.

This content is created by a diverse group of men and women from all over the world who donate their time and energy to this unorthodox relaxation technique, and their efforts have won them legions of fans. However, there is one individual who rises above the rest and is considered to be the "original" ASMRtist, even though it was never his intention to put his audience to sleep: Bob Ross, host of the long-running PBS series *The Joy of Painting*.

Ross holds a special place in the hearts of tingle heads everywhere, and many consider his show to be their first introduction to the ASMR experience. However, before he waxed poetic about "happy trees" on his wildly successful show, the mild-mannered landscape painter was a brusque military man who made his troops scrub latrines and screamed at them when they were late for work.

When Ross retired from the Air Force after 20 years in the service, he vowed never to raise his voice again. He turned his attention to his artwork and the wet-on-wet technique that would earn him a place in television (and ASMR) history.

The Joy of Painting debuted in 1983, and right from the start, it was the perfect storm for an ASMR event. Throughout the 30-minute show, Ross treated his audience to a symphony of sound triggers, including brushing, flapping, scraping, tapping, soft-spoken words, positive affirmations, slow and deliberate movements, and periods of silence that often led viewers to experience *anticipatory tingles*.

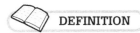

DEFINITION

> An **ASMRtist** is someone who creates content in the hopes it will trigger the tingle in another person. **Anticipatory tingles** is an ASMR term used to describe the sensation one can achieve while waiting for the next (unpredictable) trigger and not knowing when it will come or what it will be.

Ross had the rare ability to be intimate without being intrusive. Along with his quiet voice, gentle demeanor, efficient brushstrokes, and canvas-tapping techniques, he offered that ideal combination of meekness, personal attention, and careful methodology that works like a tonic on tingle heads. Ross possessed all the behaviors and traits that are central to Richard's ASMR Origin Theory.

Ross's artistic appeal and personality were the comfort "food" that kept his viewers coming back for more, whether it was an art lesson or a good nap. Even though Ross died in 1995, reruns, DVDs, and YouTube clips abound and remain popular with ASMR experiencers. In fact, it is this type of milk-and-cookies content that ASMRtists hope to create in their audio and visual offerings. They want to create an atmosphere conducive to an ASMR event, and in each episode, build a relationship with their audience that will put their minds at ease so they can open their minds, relax, and let the sensations stimulate them.

Not the Sexual Kind of Pleasure

One of the biggest misconceptions about the ASMR experience is its supposed connection to the fetish community and exactly what kind of release ASMR content is supposed to inspire. For years, those who have caught glimpses of an ASMR video featuring an incognito person along with a close-up of someone's hands or mouth understandably concluded there was something of a sexual nature going on.

However, nothing could be further from the truth. While ASMRtists strive to arouse viewers on a multisensory level in order to achieve a feeling of relaxation or *braingasm*, the ASMR experience is not about sex. This is not the kind of stimulation we are referring to when it comes to the ASMR sensation, and the term *braingasm* is a little misleading when describing the overall tingly goal of a traditional ASMR video.

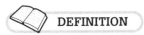

DEFINITION

> A **braingasm** is the term given to the tingle release that occurs during an ASMR experience, even though it is not sexual in nature.

Sexual release is the result of the overstimulation of the pleasure senses coupled with compounded tension in the sexual organs. Richard says this heightened physiological state of excitement during the brief moment of orgasm misrepresents what the ASMR experience is.

What an individual is experiencing during ASMR is similar to the sensation that occurs after the orgasm, when the person is relaxing. This is known as *resolution,* and it is a phase that includes euphoria; muscle relaxation; feelings of well-being, comfort, and trust; a desire for closeness and cuddling; and increased sedation—but an overall lack of sexual desire. These feelings during the phase of resolution have been shown to be due to increased release of endorphins, dopamine, oxytocin, and serotonin, the same molecules proposed by Richard to be responsible for ASMR. "This physiological state of relaxation after an orgasm is similar to ASMR," he states. "But it is not the same as an orgasm."

Misophonia: The Opposite of ASMR

Just as there are certain sounds that can lull people into a deep feeling of relaxation, there are also sounds that have the opposite effect on individuals. *Misophonia,* which literally means "a hatred of sound," is a hypersensitivity to auditory triggers that may go unnoticed by others.

Misophonia is caused by a condition known as selective sound sensitivity syndrome, and those who experience this phenomenon are not merely irritated or annoyed by seemingly innocuous noises such as chewing, nail clipping, or coughing; they actually become enraged by them.

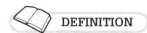 DEFINITION

> **Misophonia** is the hatred of sound as a result of a condition known as selective sound sensitivity syndrome.

First identified by American neuroscientists Pawel Jastreboff and Margaret Jastreboff, misophonia is characterized by extreme emotional responses to auditory triggers that are not connected to known hearing disorders such as tinnitus or hyperacusis. For those who suffer from it, misophonia is a very difficult condition to deal with. Not only can it affect someone's daily routine, but it can cause an individual to withdraw from his loved ones, friends, and society in an effort to escape the sounds that cause his nonvoluntary negative (and sometimes violent) reaction.

Like ASMR, misophonia is a relatively new phenomenon that has been studied only in recent years, but they are polar opposites of one another. Experts suggest that misophonia is less of a disorder and more of a physiological irregularity. Aage R. Moller, a neuroscientist at the University of Texas at Dallas, suggests that misophonia is hardwired into an individual being, similar to being right- or left-handed. It is a condition that comes out into the forefront only when it is activated by a trigger. Moller says that at present there is no known treatment for misophonia, and many patients often go from doctor to doctor throughout their lives searching for relief.

According to the Misophonia.com website, sound triggers vary based on the individual but may include the following:

- **Mouth and eating noises:** Chewing, crunching gulping, gum chewing and popping, kissing sounds, nail biting, slurping, licking, smacking, spitting, and grinding teeth

- **Breathing or nasal noises:** Loud or soft breathing, sniffling, snorting, snoring, sneezing, congested breathing, hiccups, yawning, nose whistling, and wheezing

- **Vocal sounds:** Muffled talking, nasally voices, overused words such as "um" or "ah," singing, gravelly voices, soft whisperlike voices, and whistling

- **Environmental sounds:** Plastic water bottle squeezing, rustling of plastic and paper bags, machinery, animal noises, electronic devices, tapping, and clicking

- **Body movements:** Cracking one's knuckles, neck, or back; foot shuffling or tapping; finger snapping; foot dragging; high-heeled shoes; flip-flops; and fingernail biting

As you might have noticed, some of the same triggers that affect tingle heads in a positive way affect those with misophonia negatively. In fact, some people experience both conditions with slight variations between the two depending on the situation. Both are highly subjective experiences and in chapters to come, we will explore how these sounds, along with the various practices, have all had a hand in the development of ASMR and are now being used to help people throughout the world get a good night's rest.

DID YOU KNOW?

Most people can experience a negative form of ASMR when they hear or are reminded of a sound that's inherently unpleasant, such as fingernails on a blackboard, even if they do not experience the more pleasurable and relaxing ASMR sensation. However, this negative ASMR sensation does not always lead to a violent reaction.

The Least You Need to Know

- ASMR is a perceptual phenomenon that not everyone experiences.
- ASMR is associated with a tingly feeling in the brain that some find similar to goose bumps.
- There are many triggers associated with ASMR. No matter what the trigger, though, the result is the same—a silvery, sparkly feeling that creates a euphoric feeling in the body.
- Painter Bob Ross is considered to be the first ASMR content creator.
- Misophonia is the opposite of ASMR and describes a hypersensitivity to sound that can lead someone to become enraged by even the most innocuous noises.

ASMR and the Science of Sleep

If you are someone who has trouble getting to sleep at night, take heart—you have plenty of company. Statistics say that as many as 70 million people in the United States alone suffer from a sleep disorder.

While some people use prescription sleep aids, others have sought out more-natural remedies, which is where ASMR comes in. In recent times, people who have trouble falling asleep have turned to ASMR content to help them rest and relax.

In this chapter, we give you a better understanding of the process people spend one third of their lives doing, plus information on why so many consider ASMR to be the cure for sleep disorders such as insomnia.

What Is Sleep?

Sleep is a period of reduced activity in which individuals assume a relaxed position and allow themselves to transcend into an altered state of consciousness. During this state, they are less responsive to external stimuli, but not so far gone as to enter a state of hibernation or coma.

While science has yet to prove exactly why people sleep, they do know the human sleep/wake state is controlled by nerve-signaling chemicals known as *neurotransmitters* that influence different groups of neurons in the brain. Neurons connecting the brain stem to the spinal cord produce increasing amounts of specific neurotransmitters in order to let the brain know when it is time to be alert and awake. Other neurons, located in the back of the brain, act as a shutoff valve to the others and tell the brain when it is time to go to sleep.

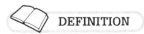

DEFINITION

Neurotransmitters are the brain chemicals that communicate information throughout our brain and body and relay signals between nerve cells called *neurons*.

There is also research to suggest that the body produces a chemical called *adenosine* that builds up in the blood throughout the day and causes drowsiness. It is believed that adenosine breaks down during the sleep state, causing a person to wake up. Once awake, adenosine starts building up, starting the process all over again.

The sleep cycle is divided into two major alternating phases:

* Slow-wave sleep or nonrapid eye movement (NREM)

* Paradoxical sleep or rapid-eye movement (REM)

Slow-Wave Sleep (NREM)

Slow-wave sleep, also known as NREM, is comprised of four stages of relatively high-voltage, low-frequency brain waves that progress from light sleep (stages 1 and 2) to deep sleep (stages 3 and 4).

NREM Sleep: Stages 1 and 2

The first stage of sleep is a very light one. During this stage, individuals drift in and out of consciousness, their eye and muscle movement slow down, and they can be awakened fairly easily. If aroused during at this stage of rest, the individual may retain memories of fragmented images and disjointed thoughts. Some people also experience *hypnic myoclonia*, a sudden muscle contraction that follows a sensation of falling.

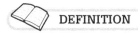
DEFINITION

> **Hypnic myoclonia** is a sudden muscle contraction that occurs during the first stage of sleep and is typically preceded by a sensation of falling. It is similar to the jump that occurs when someone is startled.

In stage-2 sleep, an individual's eye movements come to a halt and brain waves slow down even further. However, they are interrupted by bursts of activity known as K-complexes and sleep spindles:

- *K-complexes* are large waves that occur in response to environmental stimuli (for example, the whirring of a ceiling fan, a dog barking, or noises in the bedroom).

- *Sleep spindles* mediate sleep-related functions, such as combining new information with a person's existing knowledge and remembering and forgetting.

Those who are awakened in the first two stages of sleep may not believe they have been asleep at all even if, from a clinical standpoint, they have.

NREM Sleep: Stages 3 and 4

Sleep as people traditionally think of it is more commonly associated with stages 3 through 4 and beyond, which tend to offer deeper periods of rest.

Stage-3 and -4 sleep is characterized by the presence of very slow, high-amplitude *delta waves*. During these stages, there is no eye movement and little muscle activity, and it is more difficult to arouse individuals from their slumber. When they are awakened from these stages, individuals tend to be groggy and disoriented, with a feeling that they were asleep for some period of time, even if they aren't sure for how long.

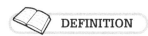
DEFINITION

> **Delta waves** are high-amplitude brain waves that happen during stages 3 and 4 of NREM sleep. Disruptions of delta waves are commonly associated with sleep disorders.

Paradoxical Sleep (REM)

Most individuals spend the first 60 minutes or so of their sleep state moving through stages 1 through 4 of NREM before entering the deepest phase of slumber: paradoxical sleep, or REM.

REM begins approximately 70 to 90 minutes after people close their eyes and includes the darting eye movement that gives this stage its name. REM is a sleep state that is characterized by muscle paralysis, rapid breathing, an increased heart rate, and a rise in blood pressure.

DID YOU KNOW?

Have you ever wondered why some people can remember their dreams while others cannot? A recent study by Perrine Ruby of the Lyon Neuroscience Research Center suggests that high dream recallers have more spontaneous activity in the temporal-parietal junction, an area of the brain known to play a part in the filtering of internal and external information. This increased spontaneous activity (which occurs in both the sleep and awake states) may explain why they are better able to encode their dreams into their memories than low dream recallers.

Although people spend about 25 percent of their night in REM sleep, the exact function of this phase is not well known. Some people believe it is the period of time in which the memories consolidate and catalogue information, while others think that REM sleep is critical to the development of the central nervous system or gives the brain a chance to re-energize other neurotransmitters such as the monoamine receptors (which are involved in regulating emotion, arousal, and other types of memory). However, what makes this phase of sleep so physiologically different from the other four is the presence of fanciful narratives known as dreams and nightmares.

In My Dreams

Dreams are the images, thoughts, and emotions experienced by individuals during periods of REM sleep. They can be detailed or vague, full of exciting emotion or terrifying imagery, and make perfect sense or be completely irrational.

Like the act of sleep itself, science knows what a dream is, but it has yet to conclusively prove why people do it and what purpose it serves. While some researchers believe that dreams are nothing more than random, meaningless images and ideas, others believe that dreams are far more psychologically significant and an essential part of our overall mental, physical, and emotional well-being.

Some dream theories suggest that dreams do the following:

- Allow people's brains to interpret external stimuli during the sleep state

- Allow the brain to clean up, file, and process information in preparation for the next day

- Serve as a form of psychotherapy in which individuals work through their feelings and emotions in a safe environment

- Are mentally generated thoughts and ideas that have loose connections and are guided by the emotions of the individual dreamer

Welcome to My Nightmare

While the term *dream* is usually associated with a pleasant or surrealistic sleep narrative, on the opposite end of the spectrum is a series of images that result in feelings of fear, terror, and anxiety. These narratives may involve real-life or surrealistic events, can occur once in a while or on a fairly regular basis, and may happen after watching a scary movie or for seemingly no reason at all. They are nightmares.

Although they are not pleasant, a nightmare is a fairly common and ordinary phenomenon that occurs by the age of 10 at the latest and then intermittently throughout people's lives. Researchers say that nightmares are a normal reaction to stress and a way for individuals to deal with traumatic events. However, they are not considered a disorder unless they interfere with your ability to function in society and the workplace.

The Lucid Dream

Deep within the realm of REM, there exists an unusual state of consciousness in which individuals know they are dreaming and are able to maintain some amount of control over the experience. It is known as the *lucid dream*.

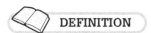 **DEFINITION**

A **lucid dream** is any dream in which a person knows that she is dreaming.

First coined by Dutch psychiatrist Frederik van Eeden in 1911, the lucid dream is a unique event characterized by seven conditions of clarity:

- The person is aware she is asleep during the dream.

- The person is able to make coherent decisions while in the dream state.

- The person tends to be able to recall more memories and details associated with her individual dream.

- The person retains awareness of her identity in the dream.

- The individual is aware of her dream environment.

- The individual has a clear understanding of her dream's meaning.

- The individual has the ability to concentrate, focus on, and influence the dream's narrative.

There are two ways in which the lucid dream can occur. The *dream-induced lucid dream (DILD)* is one that begins as a traditional dream until a point where individuals realize they are dreaming. Perhaps they notice a color and remember the adage that most people do not dream in color. They may find themselves incapable of moving their legs or blinded by sunlight and in their frustration realize they must be dreaming in order to be so helpless. In the *wake-induced lucid dream (WILD),* individuals are able to transition from a period of wakefulness into a dream state seamlessly with no lapse in consciousness. They are in control of the dream right from the very start.

Lucid dreaming is not a new concept, but like ASMR, is it not one that is fully understood. For some, the ability to experience lucid dreams happens organically, while others have to work harder at it in order to recognize the dream state as it occurs. Some people believe that the chances of lucid dreaming can be enhanced with guided meditations, sound vibrations, hypnotic suggestions, and other content found in ASMR videos.

TINGLE TIP

Lucid dreaming is of particular interest to the ASMR community, with several ASMR websites suggesting that lucid dreaming enables one to control their sleep state, go on fantastic adventures, and even helps combat common sleep disorders. In Part 2, you will examine some of the practices associated with the lucid dream, such as meditation and hypnosis, and learn how those practices have crossed over into the realm of ASMR in order to help folks achieve to sleep.

Sleep Disorders

The average sleep cycle lasts between 90 to 110 minutes in length, which means that if people are getting the recommended 8 hours of rest, they should move through 4 to 5 sleep cycles during that time. However, that is rarely the case. According to national polls, about 20 percent of the population reports they get less than six hours of sleep at night, and those who used to achieve a full eight hours is on the decline.

There are a number of reasons for this lack of rest. There are a number of serious medical conditions that disrupt the sleeping pattern of individuals and, if severe, can interfere with their normal state of functioning. Some of the more unique sleep disorders include nightmares, night terrors, sleep walking, sleep talking and teeth grinding (known as *parasomnias*). However, most people are familiar with the more common afflictions, such as the following:

- **Sleep apnea:** Also known as *chronic snoring*, it is a fairly common condition characterized by lapses in an individual's breathing pattern during the sleep state.

- **Narcolepsy:** A brain disorder in which individuals struggle to control their sleep/wake cycles. Narcoleptics can typically fall asleep anywhere and at any time.

- **Restless leg syndrome (RLS):** An uncomfortable neurological condition in which a person experiences unpleasant sensations in the legs coupled with the overwhelming desire to move them.

While some of these conditions require medication, therapy, and occasionally even surgery in order to manage them, there is one commonality. Most of them result in the one sleep disorder that is most commonly connected to the distractions, disruptions, and diversions that plague people's 24/7 lives: *insomnia*.

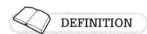

DEFINITION

Insomnia is a disorder characterized by a person's inability to go to sleep or to stay asleep at night. It is usually diagnosed by a clinician because it compromises the work, education, health, and/or relationships of the individual.

Wide Awake

Insomnia is the inability to fall asleep, stay asleep, or both during the night. It is the number-one sleep disorder of all time, is often a byproduct of other conditions, and is the disorder that is most commonly associated to the ASMR phenomenon. According to the American Academy of Sleep Medicine, insomnia is a condition that affects a significant percentage of the population, with 30 to 35 percent of people suffering brief periods of sleeplessness, 15 to 20 percent enduring short-term sleep loss, and approximately 10 percent of the population dealing with chronic insomnia that occurs at least three times a week for three months or longer.

When people suffer from insomnia, they never feel adequately rested; this lack of rest can then have a negative impact on their health and everyday life. While some people do not require as much sleep as others, a long-term deprivation of what feels normal to them can lower their energy level, depress their mood, and decrease their performance level at work and at home. According to the Mayo Clinic, the symptoms of insomnia may include the following:

- Difficulty falling asleep at night

- Awakening during the night

- Awakening too early

- Not feeling well rested after a night's sleep

- Daytime tiredness or sleepiness

- Irritability, depression, or anxiety

- Difficulty paying attention, focusing on tasks, or remembering

- Increased errors or accidents

- Tension headaches

- Distress in the stomach and intestines (gastrointestinal tract)

- Ongoing worries about sleep

So what is keeping everyone awake at night? Experts say that it is a condition caused by stress, anxiety, depression, underlying medical conditions, poor sleep habits, current medications, or a change in work or living environment. Insomnia is something that has a tendency to increase with age and often occurs more in women than in men. It can also be more prevalent in people over the age of 60, those who have a history of behavioral health issues, folks who travel great distances on a regular basis, individuals enduring pressures, or those who work on a schedule that is not conducive to sleep.

The first step in alleviating any sleep disorder is to adopt healthy sleep-hygiene habits, such as creating a sleep schedule and avoiding naps. However, sometimes the solution to sleeplessness is not as simple as making a few lifestyle adjustments, and that's where ASMR and YouTube come into the equation.

How ASMR Can Help

Science has concluded that sleep is an important component to people's overall health and well-being. Researchers know that a good night's sleep can improve mental and physical functioning, quality of life, and the ability to learn new things.

The inability to sleep is a nightmare (pardon the pun). If you're one of those people who eschews chemical solutions to their sleeplessness and longs for a more natural (if unconventional) remedy, ASMR is a viable alternative.

For example, Emily Hanson is just one of the many tingle heads who claim that ASMR videos have helped her deal with chronic insomnia. In an interview with ABC News, she said that she didn't want to have a glass of wine or turn to pills in order to relax and that over the years, she never found meditation to be particularly helpful.

After turning to ASMR videos on the internet, Hanson said she found her cure for sleeplessness. She became hooked on the YouTube content, which enabled her eyes to grow heavy and her brain to relax. She said that she became so connected to the sounds, images, and vocal suggestions that she was able to fall asleep quickly without medication, adverse side effects, or the chance of succumbing to an unhealthy addiction. "I just conk out," she said.

Those who use ASMR videos to get to sleep attribute their effectiveness to the mundane and monotonous activity found within them, which enable them to get some shut-eye. Others say it is the idea of being the center of the ASMRtist's focus and attention that knocks them out at night. Still others claim it is the sounds and activities in the videos that connect them to the pleasant memories of their past. Whatever the reason they are drawn to the content, it seems to be working for them, and many of the top ASMRtists on YouTube have over 100,000 subscribers attesting to their videos' success.

Anecdotal evidence aside, the scientific jury is still out on the subject and is unsure as to exactly why and how these videos work on the subconscious. (At least one study on ASMR has been conducted, though as of this writing, its findings have not been published.) Still, while there have been skeptics of the practice in the past, in recent months, experts have weighed in and expressed support for ASMR. Dr. Mehmet Oz has endorsed the practice, calling it a "safe and natural way for you to fall asleep without medication" and Dr. Carl W. Bazil, a sleep disorder specialist at Columbia University, says ASMR videos are not very different from other practices known for helping folks calm down at night.

"People who have insomnia are in a hyper state of arousal," he said. "Behavior treatments— guided imagery, progressive relaxation, hypnosis and meditation—are meant to try and trick your conscious into doing what you want it to do. ASMR videos seem to be a variation on finding ways to shut your brain down."

Although there is ASMR content on the internet specifically designed to help with insomnia, various trigger videos have been known to do the trick. The following are a few to try:

- **TheUKASMR: The ASMR Sleep Clinic—To Help You Fall Asleep** (youtube.com/watch?v=_qscmiLap-g)

- **Heather Feather: Binaural ASMR. "The Sleep Police" Role-Play for Tingles, Relaxation, and of Course Sleep** (youtube.com/watch?v=nuJDv4ahiec)

- **asmrnovastar: AMSR (HD) Virtual Spa and Sleep Center with Relaxation Induction (Panning)** (youtube.com/watch?v=SgQm8REqfAw)

- **asmrkitten: ASMR Sleep Healer Role-Play** (youtube.com/watch?v=2UvUjaKWBvs)

- **ASMRvelous: Guided Sleep Relaxation—ASMR Softly Spoken** (youtube.com/watch?v=K1BJlqdODBY)

- **Ephemeral Rift: The ASMR Lounge #1—Introduction—Whispered Binaural Session for Relaxation, Meditation, and Sleep** (youtube.com/watch?v=UiwRz1Ig11M)

 KEEP IN MIND

While ASMR videos can be an effective way to help you get to sleep, they should not be used to escape any underlying problems or issues in your life.

The Least You Need to Know

- Individuals spend one third of their lives asleep.
- A lucid dream is one in which an individual knows she is dreaming.
- Sleep disorders affect tens of millions of people and range from the common to the more unusual, with one thing seemingly in common: insomnia.
- ASMR content is being used to help those who have trouble falling asleep and in recent months has been endorsed by some individuals within the medical community.

Understanding Stress

It is a six-letter word that causes hearts to pound, palms to sweat, and muscles to tighten; a bodily function designed to help people survive, but one that over time has become the scourge of their lives. It can compromise the immune system, kill brain cells, add fat to people's bellies, and even unravel chromosomes. It is stress.

Stress is not a state of mind. It is a physiological response within the body that can help people rise to the occasion and meet challenges head on, but can also upend their equilibrium, compromise their health, and shorten their time on Earth. However, similar to those with sleep issues, people have embraced ASMR as a way to get away from those problems associated with stress and into a relaxed frame of mind.

In this chapter, we take a deeper look at how stress works. We uncover what goes on in the body when people are stressed, why they can't seem to turn it off, and why they are turning to ASMR videos in order to help them relax.

In This Chapter

- What is the stress response?
- How stress can affect you physically
- Becoming part of a community of support
- De-stressing with ASMR videos

Under Pressure: Fight or Flight on Overdrive

It is no secret that people live in a state of perpetual anxiety. From the moment they wake up in the morning until the time they go to bed, people's lives are jam-packed with places to go, things to do, people to see, and bills to pay. If you're like many people, you constantly struggle to balance your workplace responsibilities with your family commitments, personal life, and social activities while trying to convince yourself that you have everything under control and you thrive on the pressure. In truth, you are likely exhausted and overwhelmed by the *stress* in your life, which is a factor in 60 percent of all human illness and disease.

Stress isn't supposed to be affecting you this way. In reality, stress isn't supposed to be a bad thing at all. In fact, stress is the body's natural defense system to any situation that threatens to disrupt the status quo.

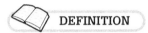 **DEFINITION**

Stress is the physical and emotional reaction to the changes and challenges that affect individuals on a daily basis.

Whenever your body feels threatened, a tiny region in the back of the brain known as the hypothalamus sounds an alarm. This alarm sends a signal to the adrenal glands, which sit on top of the kidneys, to release a surge of hormones into the blood. These hormones—adrenaline and cortisol—cause an increase in heart rate, a rise in blood pressure, and a rush of blood sugars designed to give you a boost of energy that will either lead you to combat the threat or run away from the potential danger. You know this stress response as *fight or flight*.

The fight-or-flight response is pretty important to the animal kingdom. It is the sensor that alerts you to potential danger and then gives you the strength you need to survive a direct threat on your personal being. (Your colleagues in the eat-or-be-eaten realm of the wild understand this concept.) When the immediate crisis is over, the hormone levels return to normal until the next time.

The fight-or-flight response can be a positive in your life. It can help you react quickly when an animal darts out into the road in front of your car and encourage you to avoid a situation that doesn't quite feel right. It can give you the energy you need to get through a competition and help you be on top of your game for a performance, a job interview, or when taking a test. When balanced, stress is the kind of thing that can keep you alert and top of your game.

Unfortunately, your body does not always reset itself to a normal level, and this is where you get into trouble. While animals' stress levels begin and end with their ability to survive an immediate threat, people tend to stress out over everything! Like others, you probably worry about yourself, your family, your friends, your education, your job, your bills, your health, the government, the economy, the environment … the list goes on and on. You can be plagued by a sense of inner turmoil over the things you can control, as well as the things you cannot, and it never seems to stop.

The human body is not set up to deal with this constant surge of hormones or to operate at a high level of alertness for long periods of time. When it does, its systems begin to founder and shut down, opening the door for other health problems to occur.

DID YOU KNOW?

The tension of a stringed instrument is a good illustration of how stress in the body works. When the tension is too loose, it does not make the right sound. When it is too tight, the strings can snap. There has to be a healthy balance of stress, like an instrument tuned to the middle, so the body can react quickly when the occasion calls for it.

The Long-Term Physical Effects of Stress

Discoveries about the physical effects of the stress on the body can be traced back to research on stomach ulcers. A stomach ulcer, also known as a *stress ulcer*, is essentially a hole or a break in the protective lining of the small intestine or in the stomach region. People with ulcers often describe them as a burning, aching pain between the navel and the breastbone that can last from a few minutes to a few hours and that is often mistaken for a hunger pain.

Until the 1980s, it was medical gospel that ulcers and stress were intrinsically linked. However, an Australian research team discovered that bacteria were the root cause of ulcers and that they could be managed with medication. This was a huge breakthrough that might have closed the book on stress and ulcers, but a few years later, the research took a new turn. Scientists realized the bacteria causing ulcers were not unique and could be found in about two thirds of the world's population. Why were only a fraction of these people affected?

When you feel initially threatened and stressed, the body inhibits systems that are less helpful to fight or flight. In the case of stomach ulcers, the production of mucus that lines the stomach—which protects the stomach and its cells—is inhibited. This leads to a degrading of the stomach, as well as stomach cell damage from bacteria that can more easily invade because of the lack of protection. If the stress continues, the body inhibits the immune system to prevent stomach cells from stimulating excessive inflammation. This reduced production of stomach mucus and reduced activity of immune cells are the main reasons these stomach bacteria take hold and increase the risk of stomach ulcers.

As for the rest of your body, the overall inhibition of immune cells by stress can result in other microbes wreaking havoc in other areas as well. In addition to creating ulcers, stress hormones can do the following:

- Trigger an immediate, intense negative cardiovascular response, which can increase the risk of clogged blood vessels, heart attacks, and strokes.

- Shrink brain cells over time, especially in the hippocampus, which is responsible for your ability to learn and remember things.

- Influence the level of dopamine in your brain, which affects your moods and leaves you feeling miserable.

- Cause you to put on weight, especially around the middle. This most dangerous type of body fat can lead to other health issues over time.

- Negatively affect both the male and female reproductive systems.

- Affect the health of developing fetuses in the womb, which can result in negative health outcomes for children after they are born.

 DID YOU KNOW?

Socioeconomic standing also has a direct bearing on people's stress levels. In studies conducted on primates in both Kenya and in South Carolina, it showed that dominant members of the tribe had far less stress than the subordinate members whose stress levels caused a plaquelike buildup in the arteries.

Recently, scientists have also learned that the trail of stress goes even deeper into the body and can affect you on the cellular level. Genetic structures known as *telomeres* act like the plastic tips on shoelaces; they are located on the end caps of your chromosomes and keep them from fraying. These protective telomeres become shorter as you get older. However, if you are wallowing in stress along with the stress hormones, those telomeres can shorten prematurely. In other words, stress can age you.

Dr. Elizabeth Blackburn, a leader in the field of telomere research, conducted a 2008 study on a group of women who due to circumstances beyond their control, have an unrelenting amount of stress in their lives; they are the mothers of disabled children. What she found was staggering. Although mothers of young children are typically under a lot of stress anyway, when coupled with the added responsibility of a child with special needs, on average these women were aging six biological years every 365 days.

"We found that the length of the telomeres directly relates to the amount of stress that they are under and the amount of years that they have been under this stress …," she said in a *National Geographic* documentary. "This is not somebody whining; this is real, medically serious aging going on and we can see that it is actually caused by the chronic stress."

It was a grim picture, but it was far from the end of the story. Not long after this study, Blackburn co-discovered an enzyme that, when stimulated, could actually repair the damage to the chromosomal end cap. It was called *telomerase*.

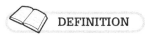 **DEFINITION**

> **Telomeres** are genetic structures that serve as an end cap on the chromosomes and shorten as we age. **Telomerase** is the enzyme that can repair the damage stress causes to the telomere, lengthen it, and slow the aging process.

In order for telomerase to slow down the aging process, repair the telomere, and improve overall health, individuals needed to make changes to their lifestyle that would reduce stress and promote longevity. In addition to adhering to a healthier diet, engaging in moderate aerobic exercise on a daily basis, and practicing proven stress-management techniques such as deep breathing and meditation, it was vital that they build a community of support including family, friends, and like-minded peers.

So as the research shows, to prevent and/or combat these problems that come about due to stress, you need to find a system of stress management that works for you and practice it faithfully. Unfortunately, that is easier said than done in a society that values those who multitask, who are always on the go, and who juggle every facet of their lives and keep smiling even when they are falling apart on the inside. However, experts say it is critical that you learn to live and appreciate a balanced and serene life in order to be healthy.

A Community of Support

Of all the lifestyle changes that have been shown to reduce stress, the two that are of particular interest to the ASMR community are practicing stress management techniques and having a community of support. Stress management techniques such as meditation, deep breathing, hypnotic suggestion, biofeedback, and sound therapy (or white noise) are at the core of every ASMR video. These methodologies allow you to be mindful in the present moment, to focus on something other than your problems, and to allow for a bit of internal healing.

While we will talk more in Part 2 about the specifics of these known stress busters and how they work in conjunction with ASMR, for now, we'd like to discuss how a community of support is at the heart of the ASMR phenomenon. There is no overstating its importance in reducing your stress, as well as improving your outlook on life.

Collaborative Care

A community of support is not the same thing as a support group, though there are some similarities between the two. When you think of a support group, you may imagine a formal gathering of people bonded by a shared experience who need a place to talk out their feelings in a safe environment. The group is usually mediated by a behavioral health professional or some other kind of official leader who ensures the conversation does not get off track and makes sure one person does not dominate the entire session.

A community of support, on the other hand, may include family and friends, as well as a cohort of peers who have similar interests and experiences and who can lend valuable insight into a particular situation and serve as a shoulder to lean on when times are tough. For example, it may be a support group such as the group of mothers in the study we discussed earlier, who come together and say the things that no one else would understand about their situation, to tell the jokes no one else would understand, and to commiserate over difficulties they know only too well. It may be bereavement support; a group of writers that workshop each other's material; or a group of fans bound by a particular love of a book, movie, or television show. It is believed that this kind of support is critical, not only for the alleviation of stress, but also goes a long way toward offering you a sense of belonging, an improved feeling of self-worth, and an overall sense of security.

A community of support can be found anywhere you can surround yourself with friends— including the gym, through volunteer efforts, school, work, and online—through reputable sites that can help you stay connected to others who may be in the same stressful situation as you. However, no matter how you choose to build that social support network, remember that it is a two-way street and there is a lot to be said for being a good friend. No one wants to be that person who does all of the taking without giving something in return. The truth is that when you help others, you tend to help yourself even more.

While it can be hard to think of others when you are wallowing in your own "stuff," it's interesting that by channeling your energies on someone else, your own stress levels decrease to a certain degree. It doesn't mean it will go away, but it does afford you the opportunity to take a break from your own problems and offer a fresh perspective on someone else's. The better you are at nurturing your friendships and not being a drain on them, the more quickly you can get back on track with your life. Learning to give and take—to show support as well as being willing to accept support—will go a long way toward reducing the level of stress in your life.

ASMR: A Symbiotic Relationship

As you learned in Chapter 1, ASMR content has the ability to calm your nerves and reduce your level of stress so you can enjoy a period of rest and relaxation. Those who experience it and know the particular sensations that trigger them say it is one of the fastest and easiest ways to calm down without resorting to medical intervention and can relieve their stress like nothing else.

> **TINGLE TIP**
>
> The most common ASMR triggers for stress relief and relaxation are tapping, scratching, crinkling, the performance of simple tasks, and makeup application. We will talk more about finding your ASMR triggers in Part 3.

However, while you may come to the ASMR community looking for rest and relaxation, what you'll discover is so much more. The ASMR community is a unique group of content creators and viewers who enjoy a symbiotic relationship with one another—in other words, a community of support. Viewers depend on the content creators to make videos in hopes of stimulating their ASMR sensation, while the content creators rely on viewers' feedback to improve their work. ASMRtists connect with one another in order to gain additional knowledge and expertise in their craft, and ASMR experiencers all over the world chat on various forums about the sensation that binds them together even if the individual triggers are highly subjective.

In a *National Geographic* documentary on stress, Elissa Epel, PhD, with the University of California at San Francisco said "compassion and caring for others may be the most important ingredients, those may be the factors that … keep us rejuvenating and regenerating." In other words, when you connect with and care for others—such as by joining and engaging in the ASMR community—it can go a long way toward your own healing process.

Members of the ASMR community would probably agree. In the trailer for the forthcoming ASMR documentary *Braingasm,* content creators and viewers from around the world wax poetic about their experiences with ASMR, as well as the community of friends they have discovered, who they may not have met through traditional social circles. Interviewees say it is wonderful to have this group of friends to turn to in times of need and marvel at how YouTube and a communal condition have given people the chance to connect with one another. One interviewee marveled that two people who live on opposite sides of the world could become the best of friends, while others say it makes them feel less alone.

If you're looking for that kind of connection, there are a number of ways you can do so with the ASMR community. There are several Reddit threads that are focused on ASMR, as well as people who connect through YouTube comments, blogs, social media, and more. Although you do not have to participate in these forums to gain stress relief from ASMR videos, for some people, the community provides an extra form of support.

How ASMR Videos May Relieve Stress

In terms of the videos themselves, although most tingle heads can't put their fingers on exactly what it is about ASMR videos that causes them to immediately relax, it is possible that it has something to do with bilateral stimulation. This refers to visual, auditory, or tactile stimuli that occur in a rhythmic left-to-right pattern.

Bilateral stimulation features prominently in the nontraditional treatment of *eye movement desensitization and reprocessing (EMDR)* used on those who have suffered from extreme trauma in their lives. Developed by psychologist Francine Shapiro in 1987, EMDR is a nontraditional approach to psychotherapy that has been shown to be effective in those who may be suffering from posttraumatic stress disorder (PTSD). Like ASMR, it is a practice that has been called *pseudoscience* by the medical community; however, its popularity continues to gain ground with those who can attest to its effectiveness.

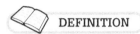 **DEFINITION**

> **Eye movement desensitization and reprocessing (EMDR)** is a nontraditional branch of psychotherapy that uses traditional talk therapy and bilateral stimulation to help individuals cope with a traumatic experience.

EMDR uses a combination of talk therapy along with something that resembles a stereotypical hypnosis session. During treatment, the client is asked to follow the therapist's fingers as they wave back and forth while recalling a painful memory. This bilateral stimulation enables the patient to lessen the power of emotionally charged memories stemming from past events.

While it's not clear how or why it works, scientists believe that EMDR is connected to the area of the brain responsible for REM sleep (see Chapter 2 for a refresher on sleep). Because it is the dream state of sleep, REM helps people cope with life's nightmares and upsetting incidents. But when people experience a particularly painful event, this process is interrupted, so they cannot effectively deal with the negative emotions. By engaging that eye movement in a clinical setting, therapists can help folks open up that process and desensitize the feelings and emotions while at the same time reprogramming the brain with more positive imagery.

For example, Eric Smith is an EMDR patient who spent decades trying to cope with memories of the Vietnam War. In the 1990s, he agreed to try what was considered at the time to be a radical new therapy. He said that when he underwent the EMDR session, it was as if the combination of words and eye movements forced him to open his mind and allow the therapy to work where traditional methods had failed.

"It would stick … It would stay," he told ABC News. "In traditional counseling or groups, I could keep my defenses up, but in trying to deal with this doggone hand movement at the same time,

I couldn't do it. I had been working on this stuff for years and within two, three, or four sessions, I resolved issues I had been discussing for four or five years with some people."

These EMDR treatments have even been known to produce the ASMR tingly sensation in some patients. Therapists such as Erin Doolittle, who have studied the EMDR approach, say that during the session, people may experience a variety of sensations (including tingles) based on the memories that are uncovered. While some are more pleasant than others, Doolittle says that the best part of the process is when one is asked to recall a particularly comfortable feeling and "flood [the] brain with delightful, delicious endorphins and dopamine," an experience that will sound familiar to most tingle heads.

However, while EMDR tends to be used for the most extreme forms of stress, ASMR bilateral stimulation is an effective option for those times you are in need of calm and relaxation.

Are you ready to try a few ASMR videos to see if they can cause you to relax and de-stress at the end of a long day? Here are just a few of our favorites that incorporate ASMR with a host of other known relaxation processes:

- **Olivia's Kissper ASMR: Piercing Pleasure for Relaxation: Binaural ASMR Acupuncture** (youtube.com/watch?v=OW0mzrVks2U)

- **MassageASMR: Reiki Remote Relaxation Session ASMR Role-Play—Hand Movements** (youtube.com/watch?v=kLhkAMPkLgg)

- **TheOneLilium: Zen Spa Relaxing Role-Play ASMR** (youtube.com/watch?v=EkRR-MI4UXw)

- **Asmrnovastar: Virtual Spa and Sleep Centre** (youtube.com/watch?v=SgQm8REqfAw)

- **Springbok ASMR: ASMR Binaural Relaxation for Stress and Anxiety, Lots of Triggers** (youtube.com/watch?v=k18I3IeboBw)

- **ASMRvelous: Guided Sleep Meditation—ASMR Softly Spoken** (youtube.com/watch?v=KlBJlqdODBY)

- **ASMRGAINS: Sleep Examination Doctor** (youtube.com/watch?v=3yBhLpXiWSg)

- **TheWaterwhispers: Suffering from Anxiety Attacks? Let Me Comfort You** (youtube.com/watch?v=hidK0FqcgzY)

- **PsycheTruth: Guided Meditation, Deep Relaxation, Help Sleeping, and ASMR** (youtube.com/watch?v=En-q519EFac)

- **SilentCitadel: Relaxation/Whispering/ASMR—A Hand Massage Instructional** (youtube.com/watch?v=OCtu2IKCPvY)

KEEP IN MIND

While it is worth noting that there are some interesting parallels between EMDR and ASMR, one is not a replacement therapy for the other. EMDR is a customized treatment program that should only be administered by a licensed therapist trained in the practice (despite the number of YouTube videos that promise you can treat yourself).

The Least You Need to Know

- Everyone experiences stress. The stress response helps alert you to immediate danger in your life.
- Over long periods of time, the stress hormones adrenaline and cortisol can affect every system in the body, leading to health problems.
- Stress can be reduced through stress management techniques and social support.
- The ASMR community offers stress management techniques but also the social support critical to stress reduction.
- Like EDMR, ASMR can use bilateral stimulation to help you potentially relieve stress.

The Origins of ASMR

Although it appears to be a brand-new way to conquer sleeplessness and stress, ASMR is a relaxation methodology that contains elements of much older spiritual and clinical practices, including meditation, hypnosis, white noise, and biofeedback, among others.

When ASMRtists create their content, they infuse many of these practices into their work to give their listeners or viewers a peaceful environment in which to slow their heart rate, block out the noise of the day, and succumb to slumber at last.

In this part, we explore the various practices that have contributed to the ASMR phenomenon and taken relaxation to the next level. You learn about the different methods of meditation, learn to concentrate on the sounds associated with white noise, and discover the power of suggestion that is hypnosis. You even get tips on how to become aware of the signs your body sends and learn more about the evolution of the "whisper" community that has helped viewers embrace a new mental reality.

Meditation

It is a relaxation practice that has been in existence for thousands of years and is used by millions to relieve stress, re-energize the body, and restore the soul. It is easy, inexpensive, and can be done anytime, anywhere, and by anyone. It is the ancient art of meditation.

Although it is typically associated with Eastern cultures, religious practices, and the martial arts, in the last century meditation has not only won the West but also the endorsement of the medical community. Experts say that meditation can calm the mind, shut out the noise of the day, and have a positive impact on people's overall health and well-being.

In this chapter, we examine this practice that many consider to be at the heart of ASMR. We tap into its rich history, uncover its benefits, and learn how ASMRtists are using elements of this art form to take their content to a whole new level.

In This Chapter

- What is meditation?
- Buddha tested, doctor approved
- Learning to let go
- Meditation and ASMR

The History of Meditation

The term *meditation* refers to a wide range of contemplative relaxation methodologies used by individuals to achieve physical, emotional, mental, and spiritual balance in their lives. It is characterized by the act of silencing the mind and turning attention inward in order to attain a sense of inner peace and clarity.

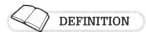 **DEFINITION**

Meditation is the act or process of spending time in quiet contemplation.

Meditation is a practice that has been around for a very long time; however, the exact origin remains unknown. Although the technique is traditionally associated with countries such as India, China, and Japan, scholars say it is probably a universal concept that was discovered by early hunting and gathering societies who first stared into their tribal fires and pondered the meaning of life.

The earliest recorded history of meditation-like practices (known as *Tantras*) was found in the Vedas, a collection of ancient Indian texts believed to have been penned around 1500 B.C.E. The process developed, expanded, and spread throughout the region over the next millennium.

Buddha's Influence on Meditation

Meditation's popularity is largely credited to a sage born in the Himalayan foothills between the sixth and fourth centuries B.C.E., who not only became the poster child for the meditative process, but also the father of his own religious movement: Buddha.

Although scholars agree that the Buddha was a real man who grew up to be one of the most influential spiritual leaders of all time, many of the stories and legends surrounding his biography are debated. What is generally accepted is that Buddha was born Siddhārta Gautama in what is now modern-day Nepal in approximately 500 B.C.E. The son of a king, Siddhārta's mother died shortly after his delivery, and in an effort to protect the boy from any further tragedy, Siddhārta's father opted to raise the boy in an opulent palace devoid of any contact with the outside world.

As per the custom of the time and culture, Siddhārta married at the age of 16 but continued to live in solitude for the next 13 years. When he ventured outside the palace walls at the age of 29, reality hit him hard. He saw the pain and suffering that he had been blind to for so long and his mind filled with questions about the human condition. After making a few more exploratory journeys and realizing that suffering was everywhere, he made the decision to leave his kingdom, his family (including his wife and son), and his "ivory tower" behind in order to live life as an *ascetic*.

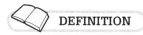

DEFINITION

An **ascetic** is one who practices severe self-discipline and abstention for religious or philosophical purposes.

Over the next six years, Siddhārta lived in abject poverty. He denied himself of all worldly pleasures, practiced self-mortification, and fasted to the point of starvation. He studied a variety of meditation techniques and followed the teachings of noted religious leaders of the day, but remained unfulfilled. Nothing Siddhārta learned could help him relieve the universal suffering that appeared to be at the very heart of human existence.

At a moment of great disappointment and disillusion, Siddhārta accepted a bowl of rice pudding and milk from a young girl. This caused his fellow ascetics to label him as greedy and someone who could not rise above his hunger. Siddhārta suddenly had a realization that deprivation hadn't brought him anymore answers than his life of opulence did. He concluded that perhaps true happiness came from living a balanced and moderate life as opposed to a life of extremes, a philosophy he called the *Middle Way*.

Armed with this new awareness and determined to find the answers at last, Siddhārta settled beneath the Bodhi tree and went into a meditative state that lasted for nearly 50 days. During this period, he purified his mind, examined his life, and battled a demon that challenged his quest for enlightenment. According to the legend, Siddhārta touched his hand to the ground, asked the universe for strength, and banished the demon forever. In that moment, an image formed in his mind of all that had happened in the universe. He received all of the answers to all of the questions that had plagued him over the years. He was awakened. From that moment on, he ceased to be known by his birth name and was forever known as the Buddha, a name that means "awakened" or "enlightened one."

DID YOU KNOW?

The story of the Buddha's enlightenment has several parallels to the story of Jesus' temptation in the desert prior to his public ministry.

Initially, Buddha was hesitant to teach. He felt that much of what he had to share could not be expressed in words. However, after his enlightenment via meditation, he offered his first sermon, known as *Dhammacakkappavattana Sutta* (*The Setting in Motion the Wheel of the Dharma*). It contained the two philosophies that would become the foundation for Buddhism: the Four Noble Truths and the Eightfold Path.

- **The Four Noble Truths:** These are centered on the nature and causes of suffering, as well as how it can be eliminated from one's life.

> • **The Eightfold Path:** This asserts that people must have the right concentration, understanding, thought, speech, action, mindfulness, livelihood, and effort to eliminate suffering in their lives.

Over the next 45 years, Buddha traveled extensively, preached his philosophies, and formed a Sangha (a community of monks that welcomed women and believed in equal opportunity for all), while remaining an advocate for the meditative practice. In fact, the Buddhist tradition spawned a number of meditation techniques, some of which we will highlight a little later in this chapter. Buddha went to his grave believing that everyone who calms their mind and opens their heart to the truth as he did through meditation can find inner peace and reach the state of *nirvana*.

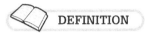 **DEFINITION**

In the Buddhist tradition, **nirvana** is a peaceful state of mind that is free of ignorance, hatred, greed, and other desecrations.

Meditation Moves West

The Buddha's influence, philosophies, and practices spread throughout the region and—whether directly tied to the famous guru or not—meditation techniques could be found in a number of religious traditions, including Judaism (Kabala), Islam (Tafakkur and Sufism), Hindu, Taoism, and even Eastern Christian movements. However, its journey West was a much slower process. Although the ancient texts had made their way to the hands of Western academics and intellectuals by the late eighteenth century, it wasn't until the mid-twentieth century that Eastern practices began to flourish in Western society. This was thanks in part to the publication of *Siddharta* by German poet, novelist, and painter Herman Hesse, as well as the first English translation of the *Tibetan Book of the Dead*. Both of these books introduced westerners to Eastern practices, including meditation, the journey of self-discovery, and the stages of consciousness.

The post–World War II era added fuel to the fire thanks to the number of Allied service members who had spent time in the Pacific theater and had personal experience with Eastern practices. Beat generation authors such as Jack Kerouac and Allen Ginsburg peppered their writings with Eastern philosophies throughout the 1950s, and in the 1960s, a little-known sage by the name of Maharishi Mahesh Yogi made headlines worldwide when four lads from Liverpool, England, traveled thousands of miles to sit at his feet and learn from him.

Although it is hard to say just how much of an influence the Beatles had on the popularity of Eastern culture and meditative practice, it is fair to say that meditation techniques were widely embraced by the counterculture, who were determined to rise above the tumultuous world they were living in during the Vietnam era. Yoga studios and Transcendental meditation centers began to dot the landscape throughout the late 1960s and early 1970s, and it wasn't long before researchers began to wonder if there were any health benefits to these "New Age" practices.

In 1979, Jon Kabat-Zinn established the Mindfulness-Based Stress Reduction Program at the University of Massachusetts in hopes of using meditation practices to treat patients with chronic illnesses. This not only gave meditation some clinical legitimacy, but also ushered in a new wave of awareness that has continued into the twenty-first century.

Mind Over Matter

Over the past 50 to 60 years, scientists have worked tirelessly to gain a better understanding of meditative techniques, how the techniques tie into wellness, and how they can benefit people's lives. There are also some who are trying to determine what, if any, connection these practices have to the ASMR phenomenon.

It is generally believed by the clinical community that meditation can lower stress and anxiety, help fight depression and addictions, manage pain, improve cognitive functioning and creativity, build internal energy, develop positive character qualities, reduce negative emotions, and combat sleep disorders. But *how* does meditation do that?

A 2011 study conducted by a team of researchers at Massachusetts General Hospital sought to explain this mind-body connection and what happens in the brain when people meditate. Using MRI technology, they studied images of their subjects' brains before and after meditation. What they discovered is that when an individual meditates, the brain does not process information as it did before. Instead, the following happens:

- There is a general decrease in beta waves, which are often associated with active, busy, or anxious thinking and active concentration.

- The frontal lobe, the most highly evolved part of the brain, goes offline.

- The activity in the parietal lobe, which is responsible for translating sensory information, is reduced.

- The information that passes through the thalamus, which regulates consciousness and alertness, slows to a crawl.

- The reticular formation, which acts as the brain's sentry, is no longer on "high alert" and is less likely to respond to stimuli and arousal.

According to Britta Hölzer, lead author of the group's paper, which appeared in the January 30, 2011, issue of *Psychiatry Research: Neuroimaging*, through the practice of meditation, people "can play an active role in changing the brain and increase [their] well-being and quality of life."

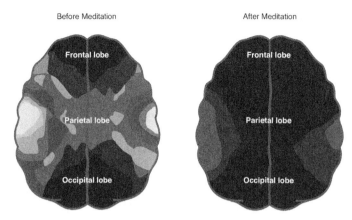

An illustration based on MRIs of a person's brain before and after meditation. Notice how much calmer the brain looks in the postmeditation scan.

How to Meditate

Meditation techniques are as wide and varied as the people who practice them. They can be part of a religious service (such as prayer, scripture reading, and reflection) or strictly secular. They can be formalized methodologies taught by certified professionals or they can be simple, informal strategies infused into everyday life.

> **TINGLE TIP**
>
> Another way to enhance the meditation experience is to add sounds of nature, such as water, birds, or the rustling of leaves. Some people assert this helps calm the mind and enables you to relax.

Regardless of what technique you may be drawn to, there are a few elements that will help prepare you and may help improve your chances of experiencing ASMR at the same time:

- **Practice in a peaceful environment.** If you are new to meditation or ASMR, it's best to have as few distractions as possible in order to concentrate on the task at hand.

- **Wear comfortable clothing.** Weather-appropriate, nonrestrictive clothing is best for the meditation process. Shoes should be removed, but socks may be worn.

- **Set a timer.** While having a "shot clock" of sorts can be distracting, some prefer to have their session monitored so they do not have to constantly check the time.

- **Stretch out.** In meditation practices, you tend to stay in one position for a long time, so it is beneficial to stretch your muscles before beginning to keep them from getting stiff.

- **Get comfortable.** Traditionally, people meditate while sitting in the lotus or half-lotus position (legs crossed), but it is permissible to use a chair or to lie down.

- **Close your eyes.** Although your eyes can remain open, closing them is another way of reducing external distractions.

- **Focus on your breath.** This step helps you regulate your oxygen intake and reduces the use of muscles in your neck, shoulders, and upper chest.

- **Practice visualization.** The more detailed and vivid the imagery in your mind, the more successful your meditation session will be.

- **Scan your body.** By focusing on individual body parts as you meditate, you can eliminate any unnoticed tension and anxiety.

So take heart. Meditation doesn't require you to don a robe, sit cross-legged on a pillow, or chant for hours on end in order to meditate. It's simply about finding a quiet place where you can open your mind and letting your energy flow.

Common Meditative Practices

Are you ready to explore this ancient art form in order to see if it can help trigger your tingles to help you relax and get some rest at night? Chances are if you are experimenting with ASMR or are a known tingle head, you have probably already had some experience with meditation, but if not, here are a few techniques to get you started. While some are more ASMR friendly than others, it's worth exploring a few of them to see if any have the ability to help you tap into your tingles or enjoy a more intense ASMR episode. For more information about the different types of meditative practices, you can visit University of the Heart at iam-u.org.

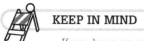 KEEP IN MIND

If you have an existing medical condition, you should consult with your physician before beginning any meditative (or ASMR) practice. Some techniques can exacerbate or worsen symptoms in people with certain conditions and produce feelings of confusion and apprehension.

Mindfulness

Mindfulness is a basic form of meditation that comes from the Buddhist tradition and is one of the most popular meditative techniques in the Western world. Mindfulness is all about awareness and acknowledgment without judgment and is achieved by finding a quiet place in which you can settle your mind, concentrate on your breathing, and let your thoughts come and go.

Mindfulness is a versatile practice that can be performed anytime and anywhere (such as on a walk, when waking, or as part of your bedtime ritual). When you are being mindful, there is no need to concentrate on any particular thread or emotion; instead, you simply observe the thoughts that cross your mind in the same way you might observe a sky full of fluffy white clouds passing overhead—with passive indifference. You can acknowledge the thoughts that pass but not labor over them or judge them in any way. The goal is simply for you to be aware of them and bring your attention back to the present.

For example, you may know you need to pay your bills; when those thoughts race into your mind, you simply acknowledge they are there but put them on the back burner for the present time. This puts yourself in a better frame of mind to deal with that and any other issues a little later on in the day.

The purpose of mindfulness is to remind you of the ebb and flow of all thoughts and emotions and that nothing lasts forever; this, too, shall pass and you are still in control of your life.

Zazen

Zazen is a general term for seated meditation found in the Buddhist tradition, in the modern Zen practice, and in ASMR. It is a minimalist form of meditation that was developed in the monastic setting and requires little in the way of instruction outside of its posturing. The Zazen practice begins with you sitting on a comfortable surface with your hands resting in your lap (your dominant hand should hold the opposite one, and both palms should face upward).

TINGLE TIP

Experts say that Zazen is a very difficult practice to learn, let alone progress in, because of the lack of instruction associated with it. Given its developmental history, it is a hard technique to adapt to an active world.

As in mindfulness, you concentrate your attention on your breathing pattern and clear your mind of all thought. In the traditional form of the practice, you might contemplate a particular aspect of Buddhist scripture, but in the more modern Zen form, this is not required.

Qigong

Qigong comes from ancient China and utilizes a combination of meditation, breathing techniques, and gentle movement to cleanse, strengthen, and circulate energy throughout your body while promoting tranquility. Known as Chinese yoga, the earliest known record of this practice dates back 2,500 years, though there have been references to Qigonglike techniques that are approximately 5,000 years old. It is considered to be both meditative and rehabilitative due to its posturing and is believed to be suitable for both the young and the young at heart.

Qigong in practice looks similar to other types of yoga exercises and contains thousands of movements and positions. The difference between the moving and nonmoving types of Qigong is the amount of oxygen that is brought into the body from the exercise.

Studies have shown that the Qigong practice can improve posture and respiration, has been known to induce a relaxation "response" (it is unclear if this is in any way related to the ASMR feeling), can cause positive changes in blood chemistry, and may be beneficial for a wide variety of ailments.

Transcendental Meditation

Transcendental Meditation (TM) is a simplified practice derived from the Hindu tradition and one that is most commonly associated with meditative techniques both in ASMR and outside of it. It is a concept that was developed by the Indian guru Maharishi Mahesh Yogi as a way in which people can detach themselves from all anxiety and rise above all that is transient in their lives. (Yes, it is the practice that the Beatles studied in the 1960s.)

TM is much more involved than mindfulness and Zazen. In this method, you sit in a full lotus position (legs crossed and each foot resting atop the opposite thigh), close your eyes, and silently chant the assigned *mantra* for 15 to 20 minutes in order to "transcend" into a perfect state of tranquility, steadiness, rest, and complete absence of thought. Some devotees of this practice even report having out-of-body experiences during their sessions.

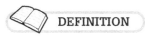 **DEFINITION**

A **mantra** is a sacred syllable, word, or phrase that is chanted in meditative practices and believed to have spiritual, psychological, or healing power.

TM is generally taught by a certified instructor; is not a strenuous practice; and, according to most experts, is generally a safe practice for healthy individuals.

Kundalini

Kundalini is another meditative technique stemming from the Hindu tradition whose name refers to the energy stream that rises from every human being. Although there are ASMR videos that utilize the body's chakras, it's not as common as other types of ASMR content. In this practice, you sit in a lotus position, clear your mind, and focus on your breath as it rises through the body's seven energy centers (known as the *chakras*).

The chakras, which are located along the body's meridian, are said to vibrate at different frequencies and are believed to be connected to people's spiritual power, as well as their emotional well-being. The chakras include the following:

- **The root chakra:** Located at the base of the spine, this chakra provides you with a sense of foundation.

- **The sacral chakra:** Found in the lower abdomen, this chakra allows you to meet new people, try new things, and enjoy new experiences.

- **The solar plexus chakra:** This chakra is found in the upper abdominal area and offers you the confidence to remain in control of your life.

- **The heart chakra:** Located in the center of our chest, this chakra is responsible for your ability to love. It also gives you a sense of inner peace and joy.

- **The throat chakra:** This chakra, located in the neck, gives you the ability to communicate with others, be self-expressive, and tell the truth.

- **The third eye chakra:** Found on the forehead between your eyes, this chakra is responsible for human intuition, imagination, and intelligence.

- **The crown chakra:** Located at the top of the head, this is the chakra that connects you to your spirituality and the infinite. Some people have reported that this is the chakra where they feel the ASMR tingle sensation.

Kundalini experts say this practice is all about awakening and that when you tune into these energy fields, you are empowered to deal with the specific life challenges associated with them.

Heart Rhythm Meditation

The heart rhythm meditation method is one in which you focus your concentration on your breath and heartbeat and use these elements throughout your body in order to re-energize. While the process for this practice is similar to that of Zazen, there are some subtle differences.

The following walks you through this meditation:

1. Begin in the lotus position (legs folded), making sure to sit up straight so your stomach is not folded over.

2. Concentrate on your breath and note the changes in its patterns. Feel the oxygen move through your anatomy.

3. Focus on making your breath deep and rhythmic (giving the same amount of time to your inhale and exhale).

4. Learn to fully exhale. In other words, exhale three counts longer than your inhale to deplete the air in the body. Do not pause before taking the next breath.

5. As you breathe, use your pulse as a guide and make each inhale six counts long and each exhale nine counts long.

6. Hold your breath at the top of the inhale and try to feel your heartbeat. The longer you are able to hold this breath, the louder your heart will sound. This will cause your heart to expand magnetically, which you should feel in your chest.

7. Master the "squared breath." Inhale for 6 counts, hold for 12 counts, and exhale for 6 counts. When you can do this for 10 breaths in a row, change up the pattern to a 8-16-8 pattern and then a 10-20-10 rhythm.

DID YOU KNOW?

Experts say that heart rhythm meditation can bring a number of tangible benefits to your life, such as building energy, steadying your heart rate, improving your concentration, making you more intuitive, and enabling you to function well under stress.

Trance-Based Meditation

This practice is one in which you are guided through the contemplative process using a series of induced calming techniques (including imagery and suggestions) that slow your brain wave state and place you into what is known as the *theta* or *trance state*. This is also the brain wave state you are in just prior to going to sleep.

Although we will talk in more detail about trance-based practices in Chapter 5, it is important to understand that in this meditative process, you retain full control of your consciousness, even as you are able to withdraw from the world around you, similar to ASMR. This technique is often used in conjunction with audio guidance, one type of which uses binaural beats to help you achieve this state of meditation (see Chapter 10 for more on binaural beats).

Binaural beats are tones presented to your ears through headphones, which work to establish activity in both the left and right sides of your brain and then create a third "sound" in your headspace. This may sound like actual music or something that you might ordinarily think of as noise, but its purpose is to help you detach from reality by turning your thoughts inward and giving you something to concentrate on as you go through the process.

Guided Visualization and ASMR Content

If there is one meditation technique that is most commonly associated with the ASMR community, it is guided visualization. In this practice, which comes from the Buddhist tradition, you assume a comfortable position and are verbally guided into a state of consciousness by another person, whether in a live session or through an audio/video recording.

Traditional Guided Meditation

Guided meditations come in a variety of forms. Originally enjoyed in a yoga studio or in a therapist's office, guided meditation began to infiltrate the mainstream and be included on record albums, cassettes, CDs, VHS tapes, and eventually DVDs and MP3 files. With the advent of the internet, online video service providers such as YouTube have opened up a whole new world for meditation guides to offer their content in an entirely new way. Guided meditations can be spoken-word narratives or can incorporate music, environmental sounds, and visual images in order to give you something upon which to concentrate.

The actual meditation itself is divided into three parts:

* As an introduction, you are led through some simple breathing techniques in order to calm your heart rate and begin to relax. You are also asked to perform an "internal scan" in order to release any stress or tension in the body by focusing on various body parts.

* When both your body and mind are clear, you begin a journey designed to improve a specific aspect of your life. This can include weight loss, smoking cessation, emotional healing, rest, and more. In this way, a guided visualization is similar to the trance-based methodology we covered earlier in this chapter because they both use imagery to enable you to focus on an aspect of your life you want to change.

* You are finally led back to a state of awareness where you feel rested, rejuvenated, and ready to continue on with your day or settle in for a good night's sleep (depending on the aim of the meditation).

The following is a sample script of a guided meditation:

Imagine yourself as a child, sitting in the backseat of a car, driving along the highway to an unknown destination on an early summer morning. As you drive beyond the noisy city, you notice there are fewer buildings dotting the landscape. There are not as many distractions along the road, and the world becomes more natural with each passing mile. You look out the window to take in the lush tree line on either side of you and realize the sounds of traffic have also faded away. Pretty soon, you notice that yours is the only car on the road.

The car makes a gentle, sweeping turn onto a long and winding driveway. You can feel that the tires are no longer on concrete and asphalt, but on soft, loamy soil. You have become part of the dense forest you admired from the main road. If possible, the world becomes even quieter than it was as you were driving and a few minutes later, the car rolls to a stop in front of a quaint cottage deep in the heart of this forest. It is your own world. Pleased by the scene in front of you, you step out of the car and touch still, cold earth with your bare feet. You can see the dew has not yet evaporated from the grass, but you can tell already it is going to be a warm summer day. You can hear the birds overhead, and you can smell the rich scents all around you. You close your eyes, hold out your arms, and breathe deeply. You know it is going to be a perfect holiday.

With the pads of your feet making soft imprints into the soil, you walk toward the cottage and peer inside. It is perfect. You can see a big, comfortable bed waiting for you and you know that you will be happy here. You walk around the perimeter of the cottage and out of the shadows of the sprawling trees to feel the summer sun on your skin. It is warm and wonderful—hot, but not too hot. You turn your head to the sky and realize it is not only the perfect shade of blue, but also absolutely cloudless.

Beyond your comfortable cottage, you can see a shimmering lake; you long to sit beside it and gaze across its silvery waters. You notice a path leading away from your cottage and decide to follow it, knowing instinctively it will take you where you want to go. The path is a slow and leisurely one, which you do not mind at all. It slopes gently and is surrounded by ornamental grasses that rustle in the slight breeze, as well as foliage and flowers of every color of the rainbow. You breathe in their scent as you walk along, descending deeper and deeper into this world. You cannot hear anything but the symphony of nature all around you: the songs of the birds overhead, the low moan of a frog before he splashes into the water, and the soft buzz of a bee gathering nectar for his honeycomb.

Finally, you come to the clearing where the lake, clear and bright, stretches out before you. You look out across it to see your cottage off in the distance—not too close and not too far away. There is a small, sandy beach at this spot. It is pristine and perfect, as though no other person has ever been there. You walk toward the water and dip your toe in to test the temperature. It is not too hot, nor is it too cold. It is just right and it is calling to you to join it.

You take off your clothes until you are down to your bathing suit and wade into the water, feeling the cool mud ooze between your toes. You let the water envelop your body a little at a time. It moves past your ankles … your knees … your thighs … your hips … deeper and deeper you walk until the water reaches your chest and you let go, succumbing to the sensation and knowing you are relaxed, happy, and free. As you bathe in this water, you feel as light as a feather with no pressures left inside. You have no cares in this world. All you have is this moment and you surrender yourself to it. The sun warms your face and the exposed areas of your body and you feel amazing. You are calm. You are relaxed. You are at peace.

When you emerge from the lake, you are refreshed and rejuvenated. The warm sand invites you to lie down, spread your arms out, and rest in its comfort and in the warmth of the sun. You lie down and stare into the infinite sky above you, feeling connected to both it and the earth somehow. You hear the birds singing around you and smell the scents of nature wafting in on the soft summer breeze. It is almost euphoric and you cannot imagine being any more relaxed than you are right now. You are on your holiday. You are in your world. You are free.

TINGLE TIP

While guided meditations are a great way to achieve inner stillness and peace, some people find the practice difficult to master if they are unable to visualize what the guide is referring to or have trouble taking themselves out of their present state and into the narrative.

ASMR Guided Meditation

ASMR role-play videos have a lot of similarities to traditional guided meditations even though they may look like two vastly different things. An ASMR guided meditation strives to achieve the same exercises as a traditional meditation, but against a familiar backdrop, such as a physician's office, hair salon, and so on. For example, in an ASMR role-play of a physician's visit, the ASMRtist may re-create the traditional breathing exercises while acting as a doctor listening to his patient's heart through a stethoscope.

Because so many tingle heads seek out ASMR content in order to go to sleep, insomnia and other rest-related maladies may be incorporated into the faux consultation before the doctor ends the appointment with assurances and positive affirmations, similar to the phase-three close of a traditional meditation.

As the ASMR phenomenon has become more popular, many of the YouTube videos listed as "meditations" have been renamed to include the ASMR moniker (though people can get the tingles from these as well). This not only allows these ancient techniques to be included in the vast library of ASMR content, but also demonstrates how one practice has impacted the other. As you will see in future chapters, there is a tremendous amount of crossover in relaxation exercises, and perhaps ASMR is simply the serenity solution for a new generation.

Are you ready to try some ASMR meditations? The following are a few videos to check out that incorporate a variety of known meditative techniques:

- **True Binaural & ASMR: ASMR (Mindfulness) 01—Chasing Your Tail** (youtube. com/watch?v=L5gKriUE1K8)

- **WhisperingLight: ASMR Chakra Meditation Healing Session RP (Crystal Cave Cleansing)** (youtube.com/watch?v=_kYdKXmw2Rk)

- **Pierre Luc-Clermont: Deep Meditative Trance (DMT)** (youtube.com/ watch?v=8ji9z0OklK0)

- **asmrnovastar: Guided Imagery for Sleep and Anxiety—with Binaural Beats** (youtube.com/watch?v=EyV474MLVos)

- **TheWaterwhispers: ASMR Soft-Spoken—Guided Visualization** (youtube.com/ watch?v=1xiVHC68-ng)

The Least You Need to Know

- Meditation is a practice that has been in existence for thousands of years.
- Buddha believed that meditation could lead individuals to a state of nirvana.
- Meditation can reduce your stress and anxiety and assist in reducing a number of other health conditions.
- ASMR role-plays are influenced by the guided visualization meditation technique.

CHAPTER 5

Hypnosis: The Power of Suggestion

When you think about hypnosis, what images come to mind? Do you picture a kitschy nightclub act in which the headlining performer waves a gold pocket watch at an audience volunteer until his head slumps in slumber and is compelled to perform a variety embarrassing stunts for the amusement of the crowd?

If so, you may be surprised to learn that in reality, hypnosis bears little resemblance to its theatrical counterpart. It is not a magic trick or mind control, and contrary to popular belief, the person isn't even asleep. Hypnosis is a trance-induced state of relaxation in which an individual is highly susceptible to suggestion. This is very similar to ASMR because just as you have to be open to hypnosis for the suggestions to work, you have to be open to the ASMR experience in order for the tingly sensation to occur.

In this chapter, we delve into this fascinating aspect of the human mind. We go over what causes people to go "under," learn why hypnosis is such a misunderstood methodology, and look into why it is so intrinsically tied to the ASMR experience.

In This Chapter

- A brief history of hypnosis
- Common myths about hypnosis
- Different types of hypnosis sessions
- ASMR and hypnosis: are they one and the same?

From Séance to Science

Hypnosis is an organic, if altered, state of selective focus and attention whose roots go back to antiquity but which became more popular in the 1700s through the faith healings of Father Gassner, a Catholic priest from Switzerland. Father Gassner exorcised the "demons" (read: mental illnesses) of his parishioners through elaborate rituals that included soft-spoken Latin and techniques that induced a sleeplike state.

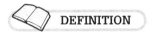

DEFINITION

> **Hypnosis** is the induction of a state of consciousness in which a person apparently loses the power of voluntary action and is highly responsive to suggestion or direction.

Getting "Mesmerized"

Viennese physician Franz Anton Mesmer became enamored with Father Gassner's work and concluded that the human body must have magnetic poles with magnetic fluid running between them. He decided that an individual's illness must be the result of an interruption in this flow, which could only be fixed by someone in possession of animal magnetism, an invisible force exerted from animals that could be used to promote healing in the body.

Mesmer replicated the process Father Gassner had been using, and as his fame spread, his practice took on a more theatrical feel. He used strange mechanisms in his rituals. He incorporated music and created a séancelike atmosphere in order to increase his chances of inducing a trance. Those who witnessed his cures were "mesmerized" by the practice and his ability, which led to its first name, *Mesmerism.* However, the Vienna Medical Council was less than impressed by his work. When they could find no logical reason for his methods, they exposed him as a fraud.

Although Mesmer was the first person to make a connection between the mind and body as a way to improve people's health, the lack of scientific understanding and Mesmer's over-the-top productions caused the process to be ignored by the medical community. It was relegated to illusionists and faux spiritualists, who used the technique primarily for entertainment purposes.

Moving Into Medicine

In the 1840s, English physician James Braid began examining Mesmer's work and concluded that the process was some form of specialized sleep. He coined the term *hypnosis* after the Greek word *hypnos,* meaning "sleep." Later in his research, Braid realized that the practice had nothing to do with sleep and that it was actually a conscious state of selective focus.

DID YOU KNOW?

In the 1800s, doctors in India used hypnosis as anesthesia in order to perform surgeries on patients (including amputations). This practice ended in 1849 with the introduction of ether, developed by Boston dentist William T. G. Morton.

After Braid, other scientists continued the study of the hypnotic process in order to assess its use in the clinical setting. French neurologist Jean-Martin Chartcot looked into hypnosis as a potential treatment for hysteria. Josef Breuer and Sigmund Freud also examined the practice from a psychological standpoint to determine whether communication with the subconscious could lend insight to a person's inner thoughts and desires.

In 1958, the American Medical Association formally recognized hypnosis as a treatment and authorized its use in the medical and dental settings; however, it was not easy for the practice to shake its sideshow reputation and skepticism remained.

In 1974, hypnosis earned even more legitimacy when the American Academy of Hypnoanalysts was formed. All of the founding members were trained under William Bryan, MD, a physician who took Breuer's work in the field of hypnosis and developed it further. He is credited with turning hypnosis into the modern, highly effective treatment technique it is today.

You Are (Not) Getting Sleepy

In order to understand what hypnosis is, it's important to understand what it's not. There is a huge misconception that hypnosis is some form of mind control and despite what you may have seen in the movies, on TV, or even on stage, nothing could be further from the truth. Hypnosis is not something that someone is forced into, and it will not work on the unwilling. It is a consensual state. In order for the process to occur and to have the appropriate results, the individual must give his permission (either verbal or mental) and understand that he is in control at all times.

Secondly, hypnosis is not a state that is achieved only in a therapist's office. Truth be told, you are in and out of hypnosis several times a day, every day of your life. Because it is a state of mental relaxation, you can be in a state of hypnosis while driving a car, mowing the grass, watching a movie, reading a book, or even listening to a favorite ASMRtist. This is called *everyday hypnosis*.

There are a number of examples of everyday hypnosis we could relate here, but one of the best may be the example of trying to read a book in a busy store: You walk in and select a book you are interested in and sit down in hopes of reading a few pages to see if it is something you want to buy. You look around and hear the coffee machine spitting out lattes, kids squealing over the latest installment of the hot new series, the overhead sound system blaring an old Elvis tune, someone asking for customer assistance in the mystery section, and nearby patrons rustling their packages and flipping through pages of their own.

Although it seems an impossible task to shut out all of the noise, you open the book and begin to read. Suddenly you no longer hear the kids or the music or even the guy slurping his coffee next to you. You know they are still there and if you turned your attention to them you would see them, but your subconscious mind has turned the volume down and allowed you to enter a hypnotic trance in which you can channel all of your focus on the text in front of you.

DID YOU KNOW?

You can't get stuck in hypnosis. Although there are some people who do not want to leave their relaxed and comfortable state, it is impossible for someone to remain in a trance forever.

Finally, the biggest misconception of all about hypnosis is that an individual goes to sleep during the hypnotic state and performs some kind of sleep-walking routine. With terms such as *going under,* this is a natural assumption, but it isn't true. Hypnosis is a waking state of selective attention and one in which you will hear the hypnotist's voice and be able to respond to his suggestions. In fact, you may even become more aware that you are in your normal waking state.

Cindy Locher, a board-certified hypnotherapist at the ChangeWorks Hypnosis Center in Apple Valley, MN, says that many of her clients assume they did not undergo the hypnotic process during the session because they could hear her voice the entire time. While on occasion someone will go into a very deep trance, it's pretty rare. "It rarely happens on a first visit. It's all new to you and you are trying to decide if you trust this … person—am I comfortable with the experience and I don't know what is expected of me," she says. "(I tell them) you will hear my voice. You will be aware. You will have thoughts in your conscious mind … It's the subconscious mind that I am concerned about."

Delving Into the Past

Just as in ASMR, there are a number of triggers and cues that help you slip into a hypnotic state. As for what happens when you do, it is not unlike sleep and meditation in which your brain waves decrease from their conscious beta state to waves that are more relaxed and open to suggestion. It is these states that enable you to regress to the days of your impressionable childhood and may offer insight into the ASMR phenomenon as well.

Locher says that individuals do not begin producing beta brain waves until they are between the ages of 10 and 13. Until that time, they are highly impressionable because they operate from the following different brain wave states that do not have the capacity to reject various suggestions:

- **Theta brain wave state:** From ages 0 to 4, people operate in this state, which is associated with dreaming, meditation, subconscious, and "zoning out."

- **Alpha brain wave state:** At the age of 5, people transition into this state, which is associated with hypnosis, daydreaming, and creativity. They remain in this state for about four or five years before they begin producing their beta waves; however, even as adults, people segue back into these alpha phases when they go to sleep and when they have hypnotic moments.

It is during these theta and alpha periods of life in which people also produce heavier levels of oxytocin, which as you learned in Chapter 1 is the hormone that plays a huge role in relaxation, trust, and the bonding process. It is believed that during the hypnotic state, people's oxytocin levels are stimulated, which enables them to relax and connect with the therapist. It is during this deep moment of trust that they re-engage with the past and open themselves up to suggestibility.

So what does this have to do with ASMR? If you have the ability to reach into that childlike state through hypnosis and slow down your brain waves in order to reprogram your mind of old beliefs and behaviors, it is entirely possible that during an ASMR episode you can do something similar. You can use the memories, experiences, and sounds of the past that you know to be soothing and calming to stimulate your endorphins, causing your brain waves to regress to a phase in which you are more open to suggestion.

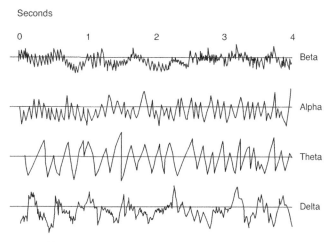

The different types of brain waves. Through ASMR, you may be able to get to the theta and alpha brain wave states where you're calmer and more open to suggestion.

How Hypnosis Sessions Work

Over the years, hypnosis has been used as a treatment option for a variety of conditions. Not only has hypnotic technique been used to help individuals cope with pain, stress, anxiety, and phobias, but it has also been used to modify behaviors, eliminate mental barriers, treat PTSD, bolster weight loss, and assist with smoking cessation.

> **DID YOU KNOW?**
>
> The success rate for smoking cessation with the help of multiple-session hypnosis is 67 percent effective, as opposed to the "cold turkey" approach, which is only 5 percent effective, and nicotine replacement, which is 15 percent effective. Even a single hypnosis session increased a person's chances of eliminating the habit to about 25 percent.

Of course, no two clients are the same, and the hypnosis experience is different for every individual. Some people may have a good idea of how hypnosis will affect them and be able to offer their hypnotist some insight that will be helpful, while others may have to seek out a qualified hypnosis professional who will take the time to find out how their brain best processes information. In the end, it's about the hypnotist tailoring a program to his client's needs.

A Typical Hypnosis Session

When you arrive for a hypnosis session, you are led into your therapist's office, where he gets to know you a little better, reviews your goals for hypnosis, and explains what is about to occur. Throughout this entire exchange, your therapist probably speaks in low, gentle tones in order to prepare your brain for what lies ahead. Once you are reasonably comfortable in your surroundings and the therapist obtains your verbal permission to proceed, he begins the hypnosis session.

Hypnosis usually begins with some deep-breathing exercises similar to the ones that are used in meditation techniques. These slow, regulated breaths help relieve surface tension in the body and enable you to be more receptive to the guided meditation that follows. While this varies from practice to practice, it might include a mental body scan to detect any "missed" areas of stress, or it might include some descriptive energy in order to give you a pleasurable state of mind where you can feel safe and secure.

Once you are completely relaxed and in a receptive state, the hypnotist will begin to offer suggestions for how you can achieve your goals regardless of whether you have sought help for losing weight, smoking cessation, phobias, or a better night's sleep. The hypnotist may also offer you detailed and vivid images of you attaining your goals so you can focus on this idea whenever you feel discouraged. A hypnotist may also offer you a *posthypnotic suggestion*, which can be activated long after the session is over.

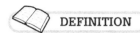

DEFINITION

> A **posthypnotic suggestion** is a suggestion made to a hypnotized person that specifies an action to be performed after returning to a normal state of consciousness, often in response to a trigger or cue. For example, if a hypnotist is helping someone get a more restful sleep, he might say "You will sleep peacefully with pleasant dreams."

When it is time to return to a normal state of consciousness, the hypnotist brings you out of the trancelike state and you are be able to go about your day, with no interruption to your daily routine.

Self-Hypnosis

It is possible for you to achieve the same level of relaxation without the need for professional assistance by employing a self-hypnosis technique. Self-hypnosis is something that is often used to modify everyday behaviors; change attitudes; or deal with the problems, stress, and anxiety of everyday life.

In order to get the most out of this experience, you are encouraged to set some goals for self-hypnosis and give those goals a high priority on your to-do list. You can write them down, if necessary, being very specific about what you want to accomplish. You then formulate the suggestions you want to use during your session. These should be positive and something that you want to work toward rather than away from (for example, "I will lose 10 pounds," as opposed to, "I will not gain another ounce"). This involves avoiding weak words such as "try," as that implies a struggle with no real intention.

One of the most popular and effective self-hypnosis techniques is called the *eye fixation*. This begins with a deep relaxation exercise, which should be practiced first before the imagery is added. In order for this technique to have the best chance for success, it should be performed in a room where there will not be any distractions and where it is unlikely that you will be disturbed. The following walks you through a sample eye fixation self-hypnosis session:

1. Sit in a comfortable chair with your feet on the floor. You may loosen or remove your shoes, but do not cross your legs.

2. Tilt your head back, stare at the ceiling, and take a deep breath. Hold it and then exhale, thinking to yourself that you are tired and you want to go to sleep.

3. Allow your body to become relaxed and limp like a rag doll.

4. Silently count backward from 5 to 0, telling yourself that you are becoming more and more relaxed with each count.

5. Stay in this period of relaxation for a few minutes and focus on your breathing.

6. When you are ready to return to your normal state, count up from 1 to 5 in an energetic manner.

7. Open your eyes.

Typically, as you master this practice, you are encouraged to add your own suggestions during the fifth step. These silent intentions must be made with purpose. They must be simple, realistic, and stated with enthusiasm and in the present tense. If desired, you are also free to add imagery to the practice. For example, if the goal of the session is relaxation, choose a landscape that represents that for you. It can be a beach, a mountain, a quiet forest, or anywhere you can allow yourself to give into the experience. This can enhance the overall experience and add a new dimension to the self-hypnosis process.

Transpersonal Hypnotherapy

Transpersonal hypnotherapy is an offshoot of transpersonal psychology, a branch of science first introduced in the 1960s as a way to integrate the traditional components of the field with the spiritual and transcendent aspects of human life. There are a lot of meditative and psychological aspects to this particular field of study. Transpersonal psychology focuses primarily on expanding your mind and going beyond your body in order to reach an expanded state of consciousness and fulfill your full potential. Although it may sound ethereal, the field has made important contributions to the research community, including new theories on perception, self-identity, and intuition.

In transpersonal psychology, therapists are not seen as experts who give answers to your personal issues. Rather, they serve as a facilitator who assists you in finding your own truth and your own path to fulfillment. One technique they use to do that is transpersonal hypnotherapy, which helps to clear the clutter from the conscious mind so the subconscious mind is more open and receptive to change. Transpersonal hypnotherapy focuses on four approaches in its methodology, including the following:

- **Underlying cause:** Reviewing the root cause of the issue

- **Habit change:** Disrupting the pattern so the habit can't continue

- **Personal mastery:** Achieving the goals you set for yourself

- **Spiritual potential:** The most important facet to transpersonal psychology, which helps you wake up to who you really are and is another form of mindfulness or consciousness raising

Side Effects of Hypnosis

People react to the hypnosis state in a number of different ways, according to Locher. She says there are those who feel extremely heavy during hypnosis and can't seem to raise their arms (if only to scratch their nose); there are also those who feel extremely light, as if they are hanging on to a cloud. Some people also experience something known as *disassociation*. In this phenomenon, the individual loses contact with his hands and feet as if they are not attached to his body.

Another side effect, and the one that occurs most often, is time distortion. Locher says the subconscious mind processes time differently than the conscious mind does, so it's not unusual for her clients to report that 30 minutes in meditation feels like 10.

 TINGLE TIP

The other side effect of hypnosis is amnesia of the actual session, but generally speaking, professional hypnotists do not want their clients to forget their session and often include the suggestion, "You will not forget about this session" in order to ensure that the memory of the event remains.

The Mayo Clinic says there are also some adverse reactions to hypnosis, such as headaches, drowsiness or dizziness, anxiety or distress, and the creation of imprecise memories, but for the most part, these are very rare phenomena and not something the average person should be concerned with.

Is ASMR a Form of Hypnosis?

Because science has yet to determine exactly what is going on during an ASMR experience, it is impossible to know for certain whether ASMR is the little sibling of hypnosis. However, in light of the fact that ASMR is an experience that can be triggered by a variety of cues, can be entered into involuntarily as well as on purpose, probably operates on the same brain wave state as hypnosis or meditation, and may also rely on oxytocin, it is a pretty safe bet that hypnosis and ASMR are at least first cousins.

It is believed by many ASMR experiencers that, like hypnosis and meditation, ASMR is something that can be practiced for more effectiveness. Because most people's first experience with ASMR happened without awareness, it may take them a while to identify the triggers that cue them into the state. But once they are discovered, they become the go-to "suggestions" that have a powerful impact on the overall relaxation process and open the door for a wide variety of suggestions and impressions in the future.

The format of an ASMR video has a lot of similarities to a hypnosis session, even if the content appears to be very different. Let's take a basic salon role-play as an example. In a salon role-play, the ASMRtist greets you, asks if you have an appointment, and possibly obtains a small amount of intake information from you. (For example... "What is your name?", "Are you here for a haircut? Highlights?", and so on.) The ASMRtist then offers you a general overview of what you can expect from the experience. He may start by telling you he is going to give you a scalp massage in order to help you relax or brush out your hair before washing and cutting it. When you are amenable to the procedure he has planned, the ASMRtist proceeds with the technique.

Up to this point, the methodology is identical. However, this is where the two practices can deviate from one another. In traditional hypnosis, the therapist simply talks you through the imagery and meditation exercises he wants you to focus on, while the ASMRtist complements their words with actual sounds and actions to help your mind re-create a familiar experience and trigger the tingly sensation that (for reasons unknown) causes you to relax faster and more deeply.

Instead of merely imagining the sounds and tools associated with a salon visit, you see and hear them. (If the ASMRtist is particularly good, your brain just might even "feel" them.) In the salon role-play, the ASMRtist may hold up the shampoo bottle and tap on its side. You may also hear the sound of the cap being flipped up, the slap of the water, and the sounds of the suds as the liquid is gently massaged into your hair. While hypnosis invites you to create a calming place where you can relax and rejuvenate, in an ASMR video, you don't have to do that. You are placed in a setting that your mind already knows and accepts to be relaxing, making it much easier for you to succumb to the experience.

If you would like to try some ASMR hypnosis videos in hopes that they help you relax, here are a few that might help:

- **MassageASMR: ASMR Role-Play by Dr. Dimitri Stress Relief Therapy and Hypnotic Session** (youtube.com/watch?v=fJ_83deKTSI)

- **Heather Feather: Binaural (3D) Hypnosis and Guided Relaxation/Meditation for Self-Worth and Letting Go (ASMR)** (youtube.com/watch?v=8nWihEWBRAY)

- **adreambeam: Sleep Hypnosis Role-Play ASMR (Soft Spoken)** (youtube.com/watch?v=4fkBZY6B1bE)

- **MissBunnyWhispers: ASMR Hypnosis Video Mega Request** (youtube.com/watch?v=32T4vpx4658)

KEEP IN MIND

It is safe to say that a large number of ASMRtists on the internet are not trained in hypnotherapy, and few would immediately equate their work to a traditional hypnosis session. While there has been no evidence of anyone being negatively affected by an ASMR video or any negative side effects as a result of watching ASMR content, there are those in the medical community who see enough of a correlation between the two that it is important to approach ASMR content videos in the same way you might a self-hypnosis session. Some individuals are more prone to suggestion than others, no two ASMR videos are exactly alike, and it is important to screen the content of ASMR videos in order to eliminate any possible concerns before using them as a way to achieve a state of relaxation.

The Least You Need to Know

- Hypnosis is not a magic trick. Because it's a state of mental relaxation, you can actually be in and out of hypnosis several times a day, every day of your life.
- During hypnosis, the brain waves slow and you regress into alpha and theta brain wave states.
- ASMR episodes can happen during hypnosis sessions because the therapist uses many of the same suggestions that can trigger a more relaxed state for the individual.

Biofeedback: The Mind-Body Connection

Biofeedback is a physiological treatment technique in which people learn how to improve their health by using signals found within the body. It is used in the clinical setting to help patients learn to relax and cope with chronic pain or any number of physical and mental disorders; in the athletic arena to optimize performance; in the space program to monitor astronauts; and even in law enforcement via polygraph to detect deception.

Although you may best know it in terms of its polygraph application, biofeedback is the way in which you can gain insight and troubleshoot your system in order to make biological adjustments that enhance your well-being.

In this chapter, we investigate this unique branch of physiology in order to learn more about how this holistic approach works; how it uses other alternative techniques to connect the body, mind, and spirit; and why it may be the key to understanding ASMR.

In This Chapter

- The history of biofeedback
- Ways the body's functions are measured
- The missing link between biofeedback and ASMR

What Is Biofeedback?

Have you ever known someone who could lower her heart rate or blood pressure simply by closing her eyes and concentrating on it? What about someone who could generate warmth from her hands like a portable space heater? While it may seem like these abilities are all part of some elaborate illusion, they aren't. The person you have come in contact with is merely a skilled practitioner of a physiological process known as *biofeedback*.

Biofeedback is an evidence-based approach to enhancing personal awareness and control over the mind and body that is used by people of all ages in order to help them make better choices about their bodies and improve their overall health and well-being. While some people come by the ability naturally, it is a technique that is typically learned in the clinical setting (such as from your doctor) and then applied in everyday life.

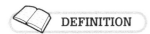 **DEFINITION**

> **Biofeedback** is a technique designed to enhance personal awareness and control over your physiological and psychological states.

If you have ever used a thermometer to check your temperature or stepped on a scale to note your weight, you, too, have some experience with biofeedback. Through these devices, your body is receiving information about your current state so you can make improvements on your condition. If you are running a fever, you may pump your body full of fluids or take some aspirin to relieve it. If you don't like the numbers on the scale, you may choose to skip desserts for the next week or schedule an extra workout session. All of these are examples of biofeedback because the information you receive (your "feedback") helps you to make decisions that will affect your life (your "bio").

Early Techniques Using Biofeedback

Although the yogis have practiced the concept of self-regulation (for example, decreasing the heart rate and oxygen intake as well as increasing the body temperature) for thousands of years, the modern history of biofeedback begins in the 1930s, when Edmund Jacobson developed a technique called *progressive relaxation* in order to ease muscle tightness in the body.

Jacobson realized there were some people who became so used to the tension in their muscles that they became unaware of it and lost the ability to relax. By creating an exercise that would enable them to systematically tighten and release their muscles, they could consciously let go of the tension from within and actually feel the difference as their body moved from an activated state to a relaxed state. The four steps for progressive relaxation include the awareness of tension, the tensing of muscles, the letting go of tension, and the awareness of relaxation. This can be linked to ASMR because of the awareness of relaxation; it is believed that the more aware a person becomes of their ASMR triggers, the easier it is to experience the tingly sensation and benefit from the practice. In fact, people usually end up identifying more triggers than they thought they had.

Another technique involving biofeedback was developed in 1932, when German psychiatrist Johann Schultz came up with *autogenic relaxation*. It was not unlike the process the yogis used and was based on the premise that people have the power inside of them to regulate their system in order to achieve a deeper feeling of relaxation. Autogenic relaxation couples Jacobson's progressive technique with guided visualization that enables people to concentrate and focus on an internal goal. The six steps to the autogenic practice focus on different parts of the body, as well as a variety of sensations, including heaviness in the extremities, warmth in the extremities, a calm and relaxed heartbeat, steady breathing, warmth in the chest area, and a cool head.

After the body is calm and relaxed, people are then asked to focus on a setting that is relaxing to them (such as a beach) in order to maintain this peaceful feeling. Like ASMR, it is not a practice that comes easily to some and does take a while to master, but it can be and has been of great benefit to those who want to reduce their levels of anxiety, achieve a state of relaxation, and lessen their stress levels.

These two practices are still used today in biofeedback therapy to help people release tension and cope with chronic pain.

Biofeedback Research Evolves

The actual term *biofeedback* was coined in the late 1960s at a time when so many scientific, social, and philosophical movements were merging into a "new age" of awareness. It was a name given to those research experiments designed to alter bodily functions that were not ordinarily controlled by voluntary methods. Scientists such as Neal Miller, John Basmanjian, and Joe Kamiya were pioneers in this field, and the three of them conducted a number of studies as to how humans might be able to use their brains to gain control of their internal functions (such as blood pressure and heart rate) and their skeletal muscles, and to discriminate among brain wave states.

 DID YOU KNOW?

Biofeedback has been nicknamed the "yoga of the West" in the book *Beyond Biofeedback* by Dr. Elmer Green, head of the Voluntary Controls Program at the Menninger Foundation in Topeka, Kansas, and his wife Alyce Green because it puts people in a state of consciousness similar to yoga and enables them to the develop some control over their involuntary bodily functions.

Originally, it was believed that if humans could master these mind-over-matter techniques, they would be able to alter their state of health from the inside out and do away with medicinal and surgical interventions altogether. It was a lofty notion, of course; however, biofeedback research has proven that the human mind does have more control over the physical being than science originally thought. It also showed that this control does have its limits and that some conditions are better suited for biofeedback treatment than others.

Biofeedback has been used in the clinical setting since the 1970s, and while the list is always expanding, some of the conditions it is used to help treat include the following:

- Chronic pain, including migraines and tension headaches

- Gastrointestinal disorders

- High and low blood pressure

- Cardiac abnormalities

- Raynaud's disease (a circulatory disorder that causes uncomfortably cold hands)

- Neurological disorders including epilepsy, spinal cord injuries, and traumatic brain injuries

- Musculoskeletal ailments, such as muscle spasms and arthritis

- Behavioral health concerns, such as addiction and dependency, depression, learning disabilities, and ADD/ADHD

- Stress and anxiety-based conditions

- Insomnia

- Sexual disorders

Types of Biofeedback

Physicians, therapists, and other clinicians use a number of biofeedback techniques to measure the physiological functions that most people are not aware of at any given time. These techniques can be used by themselves or in concert with a traditional treatment plan to improve health and well-being. The most common biofeedback techniques include the following:

Thermal biofeedback: Also known as *temperature biofeedback*, this is the most common biofeedback practice. In this technique, a finger from the individual's dominant hand is attached to a *thermistor*, which monitors the temperature in the hand as the person attempts to raise and lower it. (This method is particularly helpful in treating Raynaud's disease and migraine headaches.)

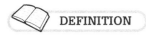

DEFINITION

A **thermistor** is a device used for measuring body temperature as it applies to an individual's stress level.

Electromyography (EMG): This is used to help individuals learn to relax particular muscle groups. In this practice, the person is attached to tiny electrodes, which send signals to the muscles; the person then tightens her muscles. The goal of the individual is to raise or lower this electrical activity through better control of the muscle group. Despite the description, it is not a painful process.

Electroencephalogram (EEG): Known more commonly as *neurofeedback,* this is a method used for monitoring brain waves. As you learned in previous chapters, human beings move through four different brain wave states throughout the day (beta, alpha, theta, and delta); for people who are under a tremendous amount of stress during their beta state (the normal waking state), it can be beneficial to know how to induce an alpha state, which is associated with relaxation. (We will talk more about this brain wave state in Chapter 8.)

In a typical EEG session, a variety of electrodes are attached to a person's scalp so the brain wave patterns can be monitored. The person then plays a simple video game designed to help her change those brain waves to a more desired frequency. This practice is used to assist with the treatment of anxiety, depression, insomnia, chronic pain, ADD/ADHD, autism, addictions, chronic fatigue syndrome, and autoimmune disorders.

Galvanic skin response: The galvanic skin response technique is a process in which a person's sweat gland activity and changes in the sympathetic nervous system are monitored. It uses a small palm-sized device that resembles a computer mouse and alerts the individual to her changes through an auditory signal. It is particularly effective in helping one overcome phobias, as well as hypertension.

How Biofeedback Works

At first glance, biofeedback has little in common with the calming imagery, soothing sounds, and soft-spoken words associated with an ASMR video. In fact, some of the machinery may remind you of something you have seen on a *CSI* broadcast or medical drama. However, biofeedback is a noninvasive treatment that does not hurt in any way. The session lasts anywhere from a few minutes to an hour, and it is in this space that the invisible becomes visible and a patient learns how to respond to the signals her body is sending her.

Regardless of the machinery involved, clinicians use the resulting audio or visual information received from these devices to evaluate systemic changes within the body. Unlike an EKG reading in which a technician administers the test but does not offer any feedback on your progress, in biofeedback, the results are immediate. The patient does not have to wait for a physician or specialist to review the test and write a report. The clinician will be able to tell the patient what signals are being monitored and what those signals say about her.

Clinicians not only identify areas that are under stress and how an individual responds to it, but they may also be able to find out how someone is using one part of the body to compensate for a deficiency in another area (which is known as *learned disuse*), as well as those times in which an individual exerts more pressure than necessary on a particular task (dysponesis). By creating a full stress profile, the therapist is able to identify issues specific to the individual so the patient can recognize these problem areas for herself and adapt her internal responses in order to reach her long-term goals.

It all sounds very complicated, but it's really quite simple. The biofeedback process is very similar to an athletic training session in which competitors practice their sport and later review the day's footage with their coach in order to assess their playing style and note any adjustments that can improve their game. The difference between biofeedback and a training session is that the adjustments aren't being made on the outside, but internally through a dialogue between the body and the brain.

 DID YOU KNOW?

Although biofeedback is a practice that is respected and acknowledged by many members of the medical community, it is often lumped in with other complementary and alternative practices that have demonstrated some promise but lack comprehensive clinical research. As a result, there is a perception that biofeedback is nothing more than a relaxation technique devoid of any true health benefits. This is an unfortunate view because it greatly oversimplifies what occurs during the biofeedback process.

So how does this dialogue occur? In addition to monitoring body signals and identifying specific areas of tension, biofeedback practitioners often lead individuals through a variety of mental exercises designed to help them shut off the chatter of the mind in order to amplify the other signals of the body and create a sense of awareness. In simple terms, they try to identify an individual's triggers (both relaxing and stressful) through a trial-and-error process in order to create the most effective treatment plan. These exercises not only help people overcome their fears and anxiety and reach a state of deep relaxation, but often they have a unique effect on the body as well.

For example, in a 2008 presentation for UCSF's Mini Medical School for the Public Series, Dr. Richard Harvey, PhD, of San Francisco State University demonstrated this mind-body connection by using a guided visualization exercise with his audience. He invited everyone in the lecture hall to get into a comfortable position and to close their eyes so they could imagine themselves at a farmhouse with a large lemon grove in the back. He mentally guided them to the lemon trees and through the process of examining the fruit and selecting the ripest ones to be taken back to the house where they would be washed, dried, sliced, and squeezed into the perfect glass of refreshing lemonade. His narrative touched on all of the senses but focused on suggestion rather than definition.

When the five-minute visualization was over, Dr. Harvey brought the class out of their meditative state and asked the group to describe the experience. The results were very interesting. Some claimed to have "smelled" the astringent as they imagined slicing into the lemon. Others "felt" a squirt of sticky juice on their hand or cheek. There were those who could "taste" the bitter flavor of the nectar and still others who could "see" the images and "hear" the sounds associated with the event he was describing. Even though there was no lemonade in the room, everyone was able to superimpose very real sensations onto an imagined event. Their minds were able to trick their bodies into thinking that something was going on.

"That's *psychophysiological* interaction," he said. "Biofeedback is about enhancing the awareness between the power that the mind has to change the physical responses or physiological reactions."

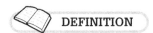

DEFINITION

Psychophysiological refers to the combination of the mental and physical processes.

This is very similar to what occurs when people watch or listen to ASMR content. They find a quiet place in which they can get into a comfortable position, concentrate on the narrative or sound assortment, and superimpose themselves into that scene. They have not lost touch with reality. They are well aware that they are not really getting a haircut or an annual eye exam or rummaging through their grandmother's jewelry box with a dear friend. However, if they can relate to the scenario, they can usually mentally place themselves in it and "feel" the sensations that accompany it as if it were really happening.

Biofeedback and ASMR: One and the Same?

The similarity between biofeedback and ASMR does not begin and end with people's ability to deeply relax, imagine themselves in a particular time and space, or mentally relate to a handful of sensory stimuli. The connection goes much deeper than that. In addition to reporting a heightened sense of awareness in their bodies and a strong desire to go to sleep during their session, approximately 15 percent of biofeedback clients have experienced a unique tingly sensation they can't explain.

Based on this piece of information, we can surmise that when a person uses known relaxation techniques to quiet the brain and harness the power of the mind to gain greater awareness into the body, it can result in the sensations commonly associated with ASMR. What does this mean? Are biofeedback and ASMR related? Could they be one and the same?

At least one researcher suggested they might be, and it's not exactly a new theory. In "Little Known Keys to Relaxation," which first appeared in the *New York Times* in February 1989, San Diego psychotherapist Randy Berkman, PhD, said the tingly sensation reported in biofeedback sessions (and ASMR episodes) is the body's healing current and a barometer for knowing when you are in a truly relaxed state. This was tested with a muscle tension monitor during a muscular biofeedback (EMG) relaxation training session, where he found "people report a stronger 'healing current' sensation in the areas being measured by the muscle tension monitor. As people become adept at overall mental and physical relaxation, they describe the experience in joyful, elative terms, such as 'I feel rivers of sparkling water pulsating throughout my body.'" Therefore, according to Dr. Berkman, tingling "is the body's built-in signal of deepening relaxation."

Dr. Berkman said that because the tingles are a great indicator of relaxation, they could be used to gauge people's progress in other practices (such as meditation, hypnosis, or biofeedback), especially if they are not sure they are advancing as quickly as they hoped. He suggests that while some people are able to experience the tingles more readily than others, it is a sensation that can be developed and expanded over time.

The idea that there is a direct connection between biofeedback and ASMR is exciting for several reasons:

* It lends credence to ASMR's very existence.
* It explains why other techniques (for example, meditation, deep breathing, and hypnosis) seem intrinsically linked to it.
* It validates what tingle heads claim to have been feeling for years.
* It proves there is existing support as to the effect "tingles" have on the body, though it is unlikely that anyone mentioned them at the time of monitoring.
* It proves that the sensations associated with the "unnamed feeling" have been acknowledged and written about by members of the medical and clinical community.

However, there are still unanswered questions. Although it is easy to understand how many people can achieve an ASMR or ASMR-like experience when focusing intently on a familiar biofeedback experience or scenario such as making lemonade, it is much harder to derive a reason as to why it can occur randomly, why triggers are so subjective, or how individuals can achieve a brain buzz from ordinary, everyday sounds. What is the missing link that connects ASMR to the very core of people's beings, enables them to conjure sensations from the soul, and gives them a rush of pleasure along with relief from their anxiety? The answer may lie in memories.

Sparking Memories

While people tend to think of the memory as a filing cabinet full of facts and figures they need in order to function or a supercomputer located just beneath the scalp, in reality, it's a lot more complicated than that. For example, if you were to recall your grandmother's house, chances are your memory of it would not begin and end with a mere description from an architectural or design standpoint. In addition to the basic visuals, you might be able to recall the unique scent of her perfume coupled with antique furniture, the sound of her annoying cuckoo clock as it chirped on the hour, or the feel of that plastic protector as you tried to sit on her sofa without sticking to it. As you can see, memories are powerful things that affect every sense of the body in subtle ways.

Biofeedback often uses traditional memories to promote a state of relaxation; ASMR takes this a step further by using sounds to trigger a tingle response when they are executed at a different speeds and frequencies. For example, crinkling a plastic candy wrapper in preparation for throwing it away may not have any effect on your ears at all. However, gently untwisting the wrapper as if trying not to make any noise may evoke an entirely different auditory experience. It's slower and lower than what people's ears are used to and therefore can affect the brain wave state.

When people take the time to slow things down and to concentrate on them, like when interacting with ASMR content, they are allowing their brain wave pattern to change and the biofeedback process to take place regardless of whether that is through sound therapy, mindfulness, or even the power of suggestion.

TINGLE TIP

As noted in Chapter 1, neurologists suggest that the pleasurable sensation associated with ASMR typically results from triggers that activate a primitive or primordial portion of the brain that we simply do not understand. While not everyone has the same frequency and most people have no idea what their frequency is, this accounts (at least in part) for why every ASMR experiencer's sound triggers are so subjective, why some ASMRtists' voices resonate with viewers while others do not, and why sound triggers can happen randomly when you least expect it.

Trying Out Biofeedback Techniques Using ASMR Content

In conclusion, while we may not know exactly what is happening in the brain at the time of the ASMR experience, what we do know is that ASMR is a biofeedback response that tells people they have reached a state of deep relaxation. It is a feeling that can be achieved intentionally through a number of relaxation techniques or unintentionally in relaxing situations.

ASMR can be stimulated by a host of visual and audio triggers that are slowed to a pleasing rate and caught at the proper frequency for the sensation to occur. It is a feeling that tends to operate on the alpha brain wave state and in addition to encouraging a trancelike period of relaxation, it enables people to shut out the noise of the world around them and connect to the very core of their being.

Are you ready to try some of the progressive relaxation techniques and autogenic relaxation methods in hopes of getting an ASMR tingle from them? The following are a few videos to help you experience biofeedback exercises for yourself and note their similarities to traditional ASMR videos, many of which are made by some of the most prominent ASMRtists:

- **Heather Feather: ASMR Binaural Guided and Progressive Relaxation/Meditation for Tingles, Anxiety Relief, and Sleep** (youtube.com/watch?v=vrSXo4tdQEI)

- **UNH Health Services: Progressive Muscle Relaxation Meditation** (youtube.com/watch?v=PYsuvRNZfxE)

- **TheOneLilium: Progressive Relaxation with Affirmations** (youtube.com/watch?v=6xUMMQI_Kjk)

- **DigitalChill: Autogenic Training a Guided Relaxation** (youtube.com/watch?v=m0e8l8dUxuA)

- **Yasmine Buraik: Autogenic Relaxation** (youtube.com/watch?v=5Lzi4T6mu0U)

The Least You Need to Know

- Biofeedback is a technique used to improve mind-body communication.
- Biofeedback uses guided visualization, imagery, sound, meditation, and hypnosis to help people reduce stress and anxiety.
- Similar to ASMR, biofeedback has been known to produce a tingly reaction.

The ASMR Community

They are the pioneers of the ASMR movement—the men and women who, bound by an unnamed feeling, blended elements of meditation, hypnotic suggestion, and sound therapy and gave the world content to sleep by. They are the ASMR community.

The ASMR community did not begin as a YouTube hub for content creators and the tingle heads who watch them. Rather, it was an almost accidental gathering of souls in pursuit of the same spontaneous sensation that offered instant relaxation. In the few short years that followed, the community transcended its subculture status, rebranded itself, and has catapulted into the mainstream.

However, its history remains elusive. In this chapter, we chronicle the early days of the ASMR community and learn more about its development, as well as the men and women who have helped it evolve.

In This Chapter

- How the ASMR phenomenon began
- Meeting the ASMRtists
- Early misunderstandings in the media
- When ASMR went mainstream
- How filmmakers have tackled ASMR

In The Beginning

As you learned in Chapter 1, ASMR is a perceptual phenomenon that is only experienced by some and rarely talked about. During the preinternet era, widespread discussion of the topic was hampered not only by those who felt the phenomenon but couldn't explain it, but also by those who tried to explain it but were often misunderstood. As a result, the sensation remained underground.

However, with the explosion of the internet in the late 1990s, those affected by this feeling were no longer content to sit on the sidelines and wonder what was happening inside of them. They wanted an explanation for the deep feeling of relaxation that occurred when they listened to someone speak softly, heard certain sounds, or watched various activities, and they turned to the information superhighway in search of answers. By 2007, the first vague descriptions of ASMR appeared on forums such as SteadyHealth.com and IsItNormal.com. It was called a "silvery sparkle in the brain" by some, a "tingling in the scalp" by others, and a "weird head sensation" that felt good by the original poster Okaywhatever on Steadyhealth.com.

As experiencers began to commiserate with one another and weigh in on the shared sensation, it became clear that this phenomenon was not unique to a specific demographic and there was a need to give it a name, as well as a community of support.

 DID YOU KNOW?

Andrew MacMuiris completed a brief history and timeline of the ASMR phenomenon on his Unnamed Feeling blog (theunnam3df33ling.blogspot.com).

A Community Is Created

Initially several names were used to describe what we now know as the ASMR experience, and some of them were used on the earliest online forums designed to create awareness and give tingle heads a place to communicate about the tingly feeling they experienced and compare notes about the stimuli and situations that triggered it. The first was the short-lived Attention Induced Head Orgasm site, which was established in 2008 but closed two years later when it failed to attract members. In 2009, the Society of Sensationalists (SoS) was established on Yahoo! Groups. It was founded by one of the original participants from the Steadyhealth.com thread and enjoyed a slightly bigger following than its predecessor, with 15 to 20 members. It was then usurped in 2010 thanks to the brainstorm of a freelance web designer and health-care IT engineer from New York named Jenn Allen.

Allen was 20 when she first experienced the tingles associated with ASMR. She said it felt like every nerve in her body had been activated and she was eager to learn more. In February of 2010, she named the unnamed feeling ASMR, established a Facebook page dedicated to the sensation, and began seeking out others who would be interested in conducting more research.

The result was the ASMR Research & Support Team, whose goals are to "better understand ASMR in medical and scientific terms, to document the personal nature of ASMR for sharing in the community, and to network with other people who experience ASMR." The team has conducted video trials and issued questionnaires to ASMR experiencers in hopes of compiling the data into a comprehensive research portfolio, which will be used to secure funding for a broader range of studies in the future.

With an official name, a presence on social media, and a research team committed to promoting awareness and understanding, the ASMR network was off and running. The original ASMR threads were archived into official forums (such as reddit.com/r/asmr and facebook.com/groups/ASMRGroup/), ASMR became the subject of several blogs and an early Twitter page (twitter.com/UNFASMR) and an official holiday for ASMR was established (Hug Your Brain Day). By ASMR's first anniversary in 2011, the phenomenon was also prevalent on the YouTube landscape.

The Whispering Community

At the same time that tingle heads were searching for an explanation for the spontaneous sensation inside them, they were also trawling shopping channels, DIY shows, and YouTube in search of something that could cause their brains to buzz. The initial online options were somewhat limited and not designed to inspire tingles. There were guided meditations, self-hypnosis sessions, natural soundscapes, and old footage from *The Joy of Painting* (see Chapter 1 if you need a refresher on the Bob Ross show). On March 26, 2009, however, WhisperingLife (check out youtube.com/user/WhisperingLife for her channel) posted a video that would change the tingle world forever.

"Whisper 1 - hello" (youtube.com/watch?v=IHtgPbfTgKc) was a 1:46 clip in which a woman with a British accent explained to viewers that she had always been soothed by the sound of whispering, and when she couldn't find any such videos on YouTube, she decided to start a channel of her own. There were no images or other sounds included on the clip, but it is considered by many to be the first ASMR trigger video and has been viewed over nearly 100,000 times.

Over the next five years, WhisperingLife posted 156 videos on her breakthrough channel. While some of them include other trigger sounds, the primary focus of her work was the whisper.

DID YOU KNOW?

When she announced her retirement from the ASMR community in her final segment on July 28, 2014, WhisperingLife reflected on the growth of the ASMR community since her first video by saying "It still amazes me just how many people love whispering. Looking back on 2009, when I made the first channel dedicated to whispering, I would have never thought that it would become so huge. It's fantastic."

Although she was the first, WhisperingLife did not remain a solo act for long. Other content creators started making whisper videos as well, and it wasn't long before their work was augmented by those who created nonspoken videos that were filled with everyday sounds. Members of this early tingle community included the following:

- TheWhisperingvoice (youtube.com/user/TheWhisperingvoice). First Video: July 17, 2009.

- Whisperchills (youtube.com/user/Whisperchills). First Video: August 23, 2009.

- SoothingWhisper (youtube.com/user/Soothingwhisper). First Video: October 2, 2009.

- Hushvirginia (youtube.com/user/hushvirginia). First Video: November 7, 2009.

- Snarkywhispers (youtube.com/user/snarkywhispers). First Video: May 13, 2010.

- Leviticus (youtube.com/user/Leviticus45). First Video: June 28, 2010.

- S0othings0unds (youtube.com/user/s0othings0unds). First Video: September 1, 2010.

- SavannahsVoice (youtube.com/user/savannahsvoice). First Video: June 4, 2011.

- whispersweetie (youtube.com/user/whispersweetie). First Video: June 17, 2011.

Suddenly, ASMR experiencers had a wide variety of videos to meet their needs. No matter whether their triggers included soft-spoken vocals, typing, tapping, hair play, or merely watching someone perform household tasks, there was someone with a camera willing to film footage of it. However, there was still something missing: a content creator who could couple the soft-spoken vocals with the soothing sounds in order to offer viewers a multisensory experience and take ASMR to the next level. It would take an ASMRtist.

TINGLE TIP

ASMR Research team member Andrew MacMuiris preserved many of the old "trigger videos" by category on The Unnamed Feeling YouTube channel at youtube.com/user/UnnamedFeeling13/feed.

The Emergence of ASMRtists

As you learned in Chapter 1, an ASMRtist is an individual who creates video and/or audio content specifically designed to trigger the tingly sensation associated with the ASMR phenomenon. While there are a number of sounds, images, and suggestions that can trigger the ASMR feeling, the ASMRtist typically uses a combination of these triggers in hopes of producing the euphoric sensation within others.

It is next to impossible to know with any certainty who was the first deliberate ASMRtist. There were a number of content creators willing to whisper at their viewers, play with a Rubik's Cube, shuffle cards, or tap blocks of wood together, but no one called themselves an ASMRtist because the name hadn't been invented. Instead, they were still going by the term *whisper community*, after the whisper videos that could trigger the tingly sensation. However, as the ASMR term became more well known, their numbers grew exponentially, and by 2011, the ASMRtist index list contained 500 names, including the first superstar of the ASMR community: Maria "GentleWhispering."

With more than 275,000 subscribers and clips ranging from whispers, to sound assortments, to show-and-tell sessions, to role-plays, Maria "GentleWhispering" was the first ASMR superstar and continues to be an inspiration to other ASMRtists.

In her video "Draw My Life," Maria "GentleWhispering" said that in order to find some peace and tranquility, she began listening to guided meditations, and then whisper videos. Eventually, she started listening to what she called "tingle videos," which led her to the ASMR community. On February 24, 2011, she joined YouTube and on June 3, 2011, she published her first video, in which she whispered in English and Russian while flipping through a magazine.

 DID YOU KNOW?

Maria "GentleWhispering" later published one of her most popular videos, a 3D selection of sounds that has been viewed over 6 million times (as of this writing) and remains a fan favorite among tingle heads. It includes a soft-spoken narrative, wooden brush sounds, a scalp massage, and a shoulder rub. You can find a link to the video in the following list.

Maria "GentleWhispering"'s story, charm, and talent for inventive content creation led her to become one of the leading ASMRtists on the web and an inspiration to many other notable names. Viewers resonated with her work and life experiences and were eager to pick up their camera phones and try their hands at creating videos as a way to give back to Maria "GentleWhispering" and other early ASMRtists who had given them so much.

You can check out some of the best-loved videos of Maria "GentleWhispering" at the following links:

- **Oh Such a Good 3D-Sound ASMR Video** (youtube.com/watch?v=RVpfHgC3ye0)

- **Eye Gazing, Ear-to-Ear Blowing, Head Massagers** (youtube.com/watch?v=_haPLEHgh8Y)

- **ASMR Paradise Lab** (youtube.com/watch?v=VJ6IWr_YNuA)

- **Russian Whisper** (youtube.com/watch?v=z1uqwLioe0M)

- **Relaxing/ASMR 3D Sound Haircut** (youtube.com/watch?v=TgpaytdDIaA)

Maria "GentleWhispering"'s story is not uncommon, as many members of the original "whisper community" began to segue into what is traditionally thought of as ASMR content today: something that couples whispers with a variety of sounds, images, or experiences. In fact, once ASMR was given its name in 2010, many of the early whisperers began including it in their titles and video descriptions to give their fans an easier search term.

The Buzz Builds

As more people learned about ASMR and joined the community, either as content creators or viewers, there became a desire to get ASMR out of the shadows and into the spotlight so that more people could be helped, and the scientific community might sit up and take notice of the phenomenon and begin to look at it more carefully.

ASMR in the Media

In June 2011, an unknown individual began an ASMR Wikipedia page (en.wikipedia.org/wiki/Autonomous_sensory_meridian_response). Jenn Allen contributed much of the content that appeared on the original site, but three months later administrators shut down the ASMR page for reasons that were never fully explained but seemed based on the fact that there was a lack of scientific evidence to support it. This enraged the community, who pointed out that Wikipedia had pages devoted to God and other subjects that were largely a matter of opinion, personal experience, or faith. Why not ASMR? (The ASMR Wikipedia page was later reinstated around November 2012 and remains active on the information hub.)

DID YOU KNOW?

Devon King, the person who compared ASMR to "Spidey senses" in Chapter 1, is responsible for the return of the ASMR Wikipedia page.

Later that same year, the ASMR phenomenon garnered its first media exposure when someone known only as "dannyboi965" from KRBZ in Kansas City posted a call-out query on an ASMR subreddit looking for an ASMR-experiencer who was willing to be interviewed on air. "Tora_Tora" volunteered and the interview was conducted on September 21 (kcradiogod.com/buzz/ABFMB/asmr0921.mp3). While it did give ASMR its first media exposure, many in the community felt that the radio personalities treated the subject callously, focusing too much on the supposed sexual aspect of the sensation and even calling the volunteer tingle head a "freak" at the end of the show.

Thankfully, the untoward comments did not stop the momentum. In February 2013, Nicholas Tufnell penned an article on ASMR for the Huffington Post UK (huffingtonpost.co.uk/nicholas-tufnell/asmr-orgasms-for-your-brain_b_1297552.html). As an ASMR experiencer himself, he presented a fair piece on the sensation, as well as how he has used it to combat his own insomnia. Interest in ASMR then continued to grow and thrive such that ASMRtist Chris "WhisperingWeaver" Javier established an ASMR Radio website (asmr.fm) and determined that the station would launch its first broadcast on April 9, the first International ASMR Day.

International ASMR Day was conceived of in March 2012 by Ilse "TheWaterwhispers" Blansert, Kelly "MsAutumnRed," Jennifer "AppreciateASMR," and viewer Wayne Booker, who mused during a Facebook chat that it would be nice to have a day set aside for ASMR awareness. Although Jenn Allen's "Hug Your Brain Day" was still in existence, they felt that ASMR had positively changed so many people's lives in such a short period of time that they contacted Maria "GentleWhispering" and several other ASMRtists to put together another day to celebrate ASMR.

The purpose of International ASMR Day is to do the following:

- Enable content creators and viewers to meet in person and to share their ASMR experiences

- Allow content creators and viewers to spread awareness about the ASMR phenomenon

- Give tingle heads a day around which to organize future ASMR conventions and gatherings

- Celebrate the feeling that is ASMR

In her 2013 video explaining the International ASMR Day celebration (youtube.com/watch?v=naJubm95jXM&feature=youtu.be), Maria "GentleWhispering" said the event was created to unite the community more and to have a day to celebrate the ASMR experience, as well as those content creators who film video segments to promote it.

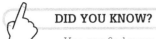

DID YOU KNOW?

You can find more about International ASMR Day on Facebook at facebook.com/InternationalAsmrDay.

ASMR's Spokeswoman: Ilse Blansert

Ilse Blansert, known as TheWaterwhispers to her fans, discovered the ASMR community in 2011. At the time, she was cramming for exams, working on several projects at once, and suffering from a lot of sleepless nights. Though she had used guided meditation tapes in the past, she had become immune to them, she found sleeping pills were no longer effective, and she was desperate for some rest.

After remembering how she used to get a warm, fuzzy feeling when she used to watch Bob Ross or when her grandmother sang lullabies while stroking her hands, she began to look for "relaxing voices" on the internet. Not only did she find old footage of Ross, but she also found a woman who gently welcomed her to a relaxing day at a virtual spa. It put her right to sleep.

"When I woke up I realized that the video had a strange word in it: ASMR. I'd never heard of it before so I looked it up. After reading the definition … I couldn't believe it. That's exactly what I've been feeling for decades and there are other people who feel this sensation, too!" she said.

After some personal setbacks, Blansert turned to the ASMR community for support and eventually decided to make a video in order to thank those who had helped her get through the tough times.

It didn't take long for her star to rise within the community. She not only became one of the first ASMRtists to accept requests from viewers, but she was also the first to offer premium-level subscriptions through her website and live Skype sessions. When her fans asked where they could send a financial contribution in support of her work, she also became one of the first ASMRtists to set up a PayPal account.

In October 2012, she became part of the ASMR community's second chance to appear on broadcast media. This time, the event took place in Europe on the Dutch television program *De Wereld Draait Door* (*The World Keeps Turning*). Blansert and another content creator, Jolien "Relaxingsounds92," appeared on the show to explain to the host what ASMR tingles are and why they make content to stimulate it.

Unlike the previous interview, the hosts were genuinely curious about the phenomenon, and even though some good-natured humor was involved, the ladies each had the opportunity to showcase some of their favorite content creators and demonstrate their skills. Blansert played with coffee beans in a plastic sack, while Jolien tapped, scratched, and crinkled for the host.

> **TINGLE TIP**
>
> Ilse Blansert's personal ASMR triggers can be found on her hour-long video "8 Different ASMR Triggers" published January 13, 2013. It includes hand and camera brushing, ear-to-ear whispering, scalp massage, and soft-spoken accents. You can see it at youtube.com/watch?v=EmR_3pj8MWw.

"It was such a shock to be invited on a Dutch TV show to talk … It's really amazing to me that the media approached us and we were very fortunate that we got the chance to explain ASMR," Blansert said on her channel.

ASMR continued to create a buzz throughout 2013, with mentions in magazines such as *Time*, but awareness exploded in 2014 when an article about it appeared in the February edition of *O Magazine*. While several ASMRtists were alluded to, Blansert's channel was mentioned by name. Not since Maria had one name been so synonymous with the ASMR community, and it's not a distinction that she enjoys.

Although she has been featured in a number of articles, radio shows, and television segments about ASMR, she said she has never participated in an interview to promote herself or her channel.

"ASMR has always been about the community, a community of wonderful people who have always been supportive of one another and willing to work together," she said. "I might be the ASMRtist who has been chosen to speak and to appear on camera, but for me it's all about the community as a whole and helping people get to sleep at night."

Coming Soon to the Big Screen

With so much interest in ASMR, it seems only natural that documentary filmmakers find it an irresistible subject to explore, and there have been a lot of projects in the works that hope to bring ASMR even more out into the open. The following are some of the films on ASMR that are complete or in progress:

Tingly Sensation: The ASMR Story: "After securing funding for the project in August 2013, filmmaker Kate Mull has been traveling the globe meeting with ASMR experiencers, content creators, and students conducting research on ASMR, as well as physicians who have been examining the phenomenon from a clinical point of view. Throughout her work on the film, she has said that she has found a number of broader and more in-depth aspects to the ASMR phenomenon (not unlike we did), and she is excited to share them with a wider audience soon. To learn more about this film and read updates, you can visit Mull's Kickstarter site at kickstarter. com/projects/tinglysensation/tingly-sensation-documentary-film.

ASMR—A Story of Relaxation: This English and Dutch minidocumentary was created in May 2014 by Jordan De Deken, a student filmmaker with Rits School of the Arts in Brussels, Belgium. De Deken is an ASMR experiencer who was eager to make ASMR the subject of his second solo production. The piece is a compilation of existing ASMR coverage, as well as interviews with ASMRtists, such as MassageASMR, EvyWhispers, and TheOneLilium. In the video's description, De Deken said he hopes that his piece sparks even more interest in the sensation that has done a lot to make his life brighter and better. He also hopes it will inspire others to see the positive side effects of ASMR. The featurette can be seen at youtube.com/watch?v=8ec9r6lX_VE.

Braingasm: Directed by Toronto filmmaker Lindsay Ragone, this piece (currently in production) centers around the scientific aspects of ASMR, as well as how the ASMR community has evolved in the few short years it has been in existence. Like Mull, Ragone has traveled the world meeting with content creators, researchers, and viewers and is excited to bring the film to the masses. Teaser trailers for the documentary promise a tantalizing glimpse into the lives of the ASMRtists (who are a unique collection of globally scattered BFFs), as well as the viewers, who say that these content creators help them feel a little less alone in the world. For more information, visit braingasm-film.com.

DID YOU KNOW?

For the first planned ASMR documentary, which mentioned in a post on the Unnamed Feeling blog, an ASMR experiencer and filmmaker from the UK was planning to create a documentary on the ASMR community. Tingle heads and content creators were encouraged to find out more about the project through the ASMR Facebook Group page, but it is unclear whether the project got off the ground, if it is still in production, or has ever been completed.

The Least You Need to Know

- The first "whispers" of ASMR began in 2007, when descriptions of the experience began to appear in online forums.
- ASMR went through a number of names before being christened in 2010 by Jenn Allen.
- Maria "GentleWhispering" is considered to be one of the most influential ASMRtists.
- As interest in ASMR grew, so, too, did its notoriety. In the past few years it has been featured in many mainstream media outlets.
- Several feature-length documentaries are in the works to help bring more awareness to ASMR.

PART 3

Finding Your Triggers

Identifying ASMR triggers is a highly subjective process that requires a lot of trial and error on the part of the person in search of the sensation. A sound or role-play that causes one person's mind to melt may do nothing for someone else, and an ASMRtist who has thousands of fans on the internet may not have the voice necessary to cause some people's brains to buzz.

Tingle heads typically sample a wide variety of voices, visuals, and sounds before finding the videos that work for them. They begin with things they know have worked in the past and try to find a video that hits the perfect pitch and frequency to trigger the senses.

Are you ready to tap into your tingles? In this part, we discuss the typical triggers reported by those who experience ASMR. You may even discover that after finding a few good ASMRtists, you have more triggers than you ever thought possible!

CHAPTER 8

What Causes You to Tingle

If you were to ask veteran tingle heads about their ASMR triggers, chances are they could tell you all about the sounds, images, and scenarios that never fail to put them into a state of slumber; the ASMRtists they like; and their "go-to" videos. It's a great place to start, but how do you know what will actually work for *you?*

You don't. There is no formula for generating the ASMR sensation. No two tingle heads are exactly alike, and there is no guarantee their triggers will have an effect on you at all. In order to find your triggers, you must revisit the past, explore the senses, and engage in the trial-and-error process.

In this chapter, we put you in the right mind-set in hopes that you can identify things that will cause your brain to buzz and reach a state of inner peace and relaxation.

In This Chapter

- Using empathy to identify your triggers
- Exploring the inner child in you
- How your number of triggers can grow
- What is ASMR immunity, and does anyone have it?

Making the Connection with Empathy

As you learned in Chapter 7, the ability to experience the ASMR sensation is intrinsically tied to your memories and your ability to superimpose your thoughts, feelings, and senses onto a described event, idea, or object. In short, you must be able to *empathize* with it.

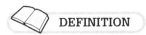 **DEFINITION**

Empathy is the way in which individuals project their senses onto another experience in order to understand it on a cognitive level.

Empathy is an important component to the overall ASMR experience. When you are offered a particular visual trigger or series of visual triggers, your ability to empathize or project your senses onto those triggers enables you to discern the stimuli in order to formulate an appropriate physical and emotional response. The more you can connect and empathize with a particular trigger, the stronger the ASMR reaction you will have to that triggering event.

Empathy is not the same thing as sympathy. Whereas sympathy is a general acknowledgment of your feelings not based in personal experience, empathy implies a deeper and more personal connection to the situation at hand.

For example, if someone has lost a spouse but you have never been widowed, you cannot say "I know how you feel" because you don't—you can't empathize. However, you can say "I know you must be heartbroken, sad, devastated," and so on because those are logical and appropriate expressions of sympathy.

ASMR triggers have a similar dichotomy. Everyone has those triggers they sympathize with even if they do not experience them on a personal level. While most tingle heads can acknowledge that watching Bob Ross paint is a well-known ASMR visual trigger, not everyone achieves the ASMR sensation from it. Those who have experienced tingles watching Ross paint can empathize with the event, while those who haven't can only sympathize with the idea. In order to find those events you empathize with, you must go back to the beginning and look for those actions and events that caused you to fall into a relaxed, happy state without even trying.

You must also consider your sensory style, or the primary way in which your brain tends to gather information, in order to engage your empathy and potentially trigger your tingles. The three traditional sensory styles include the following:

- **Watchers:** These types of people tend to notice details and are often triggered when they see someone interacting with objects in a visually pleasing way.

- **Listeners:** These individuals like to talk and love sound. They are often triggered by various noises and vocal timbres.

- **Touchers:** These people are fascinated with the physicality of objects (for example, texture, shape, size, feel, and so on). They also tend to talk with their hands.

Although you use aspects of all three categories at various points in your life, you most likely tend to favor one method over the other two. By knowing your favored style, you may begin to find patterns in the kinds of events that gave you the deepest sense of peace, tranquility, and maybe even a tingle or two.

Finding Your Inner Child

An overwhelming number of tingle heads can track their early ASMR experiences back to specific events in their childhood. In October 2014, we conducted an informal Facebook poll in which we asked our readers to tell us how old they were when they first felt the ASMR phenomenon and under what circumstances. The results were staggering. Out of the first 100 people to respond with a specific age, a whopping 93 percent said their first ASMR experience occurred prior to the age of 10.

Those who reported their first ASMR episode occurring between the ages of 0 and 4 described experiences largely focused on personal attention (for example, hair brushing, rocking, patting, ear play, and so on). For the most part, these events were designed to be soothing in nature and usually were induced by a close family member, such as a mother or grandmother. ASMR experiences that happened to respondents between the ages of 5 to 10 were far more unintentional, triggered by people outside the immediate family, and not always caused by personal contact. (Those first-time ASMR events that occurred beyond the age of 10 were generally in line with the previous category and may happen later due to minor developmental delays.)

Based on our poll, the top five most popular first-time ASMR experiences respondents reported were the following:

- Teachers' voices, especially if they whispered

- Hair play, including scalp checks, haircuts, braiding, and brushing

- Sounds associated with actions, such as unwrapping a package, clicking blocks, crinkling candy wrappers, and so on

- Art and writing sounds, including watching Bob Ross, painting, sketching, drawing, and so on

- Random touches, such as tracing on one's back, hand massages, or even the "Light As a Feather, Stiff As a Board" game

Regardless of how it first happened, it resulted in a feeling that was hard to forget and even harder to replicate. In fact, many people who hear about ASMR connect it with an event from their past but often admit they have lost touch with the sensation over the years. There are a number of reasons this could have happened. Perhaps the sensation happened infrequently enough that they didn't recognize it at the time. Perhaps other sensory issues corrupted the ASMR response, such as a touch not being as light, a voice not resonating at the same frequency, or an action sound not being as deliberate or careful. Perhaps the situations used to produce the ASMR sensation ebbed over time and eventually the memory of it faded as well.

If you fall into any of these categories, don't worry! Your tingles probably aren't gone forever. You just need to connect with your *inner child* in order to reclaim the ASMR sensation inside of you.

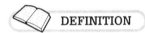 **DEFINITION**

The **inner child** is the aspect of a person's psyche and consciousness that is connected to and retains the feelings and carefree emotions of the past.

The inner child is the aspect of the consciousness that is naturally innocent, playful, and uncomplicated and whose approach to life is simple and straightforward. While it is a concept normally associated with healing the pain of the past, it is also a state of being that can put you on the road to your ASMR future.

Exploring the Past

In order to touch base with your triggers, it's important you think back on your earliest memories that you can consciously recall. Usually these are fragmented, have no context, and focus on feelings rather than actual events. You may not know where you were or what you were doing at the time, but you know that you were content in the moment. Maybe you recall sitting on a beach wiggling your toes in the cool white sand or lying on a bed getting ready for a nap and listening to the hypnotic sound of the ceiling fan above you. Perhaps you recall the gentle sound of your mother reading you a bedtime story in hushed tones until you could no longer stay awake.

Even if you can't recall them or didn't experience any tingles at the time, these events can help you pinpoint the feelings and sensations that placed you in a feeling of total relaxation. That feeling is key to the ASMR experience. When you explore the emotions and sensations that appealed to your inner child—those moments in which you were happy, relaxed, free and without a care in the world—you open your mind to the possibility of rekindling the connections on a multisensory and physiological level.

Tapping Into the Theta and Alpha Parts of You

As you learned in Chapter 5, from the time you are born until around the age of 4, you exist in a blissfully stress-free theta state of existence. You are not afraid to say what you want, try something new, or find fascination with the mundane. Although the things you enjoyed way back when may not have the same appeal for you today, it is partially because you were operating at a different brain wave state than you do now.

 TINGLE TIP

In order to start triggering your ASMR tingles, you need to tap into the events of your childhood that you found deliciously relaxing even if no one else would understand them. Refrain from judging yourself. After all, ASMR is extremely personal and, generally speaking, no one will judge you on what triggers the ASMR sensation for you. Forget the world around you and allow your mind to connect with the sights, sounds, and events of the past and try to re-create the feelings you experienced at the time they occurred.

From the age of 5 to around 9, you then move into the alpha brain wave state. As we learned even through our informal poll, this is an incredibly important time in ASMR development. During this period of time, your episodes of ASMR tend to move beyond your parents and yourself and can be triggered by others. It also tends to be when that first recognized tingle experience occurs and is centered on a situation that might not make sense to anyone else. In fact, if you have ever tried to explain the phenomenon to someone at the time, you might have gotten a few strange looks.

Chelsea Fagan is typical of an alpha phase ASMR experiencer. Fagan is a blogger at the ThoughtCatalog.com who says that when she was a little girl, she used to watch as the kid who sat across from her in school doodled on a piece of paper. She would become so mesmerized by the scratch of the pencil lead as it moved back and forth across the page that she would forget what was happening in class.

"I remember if the teacher would read a book softly to the class, every time she turned the corner of the page (with that sort of squeaky, glossy-page-against-fingers sound), I would again fall into an almost dreamlike state. I thought, at the time, that there must be something wrong with me. I always felt so weird and that if I told other kids, they would make fun of me," she wrote.

Fagan said it's not surprising that so many tingle heads do not talk about their experiences and if someone ever found a bookmarked folder on their computer full of ASMR triggers, who knows what they might conclude?

Luckily, she doesn't have to explain herself to us. We totally get it. We know that she wasn't crushing on her teacher just because she liked the sound of her voice and the way she turned the page. We also know that she didn't have a thing for graphite or the boy across the aisle. She was simply soothed by the sound he made with his pencil. Chances are if another kid had tried to replicate the same action, it wouldn't have had the same effect on her.

What is it about this phase of people's lives that causes them to become more aware of the ASMR experience? While research has not been conducted to conclusively answer this question, as you learned in Chapter 5, it is the brain wave state when you are most alert, impressionable, and easily influenced. It is the brain wave state that hypnotists try to achieve with their clients so that their suggestions will "stick."

Therefore, it is critical you let go of your adult hesitations and leave all judgment and criticism at the door if you want to trigger potential tingles. You must embrace that little kid who used to watch ceiling fans for fun, waste hours wriggling her toes in the sand, find secret delight in the sound of her mother's voice, or be soothed by the sound of pencil on paper.

DID YOU KNOW?

If you are one of those who did not experience ASMR until the age of 11 or 12, don't worry. Experts say people only begin to transition into their beta brain wave state at the age of 11, but there is plenty of that kid-level alpha state still left within. If you fall into this category, there is nothing abnormal about you at all.

The Late Bloomer

Naturally, not everyone who experiences ASMR does so by the time they reach puberty. We know a lot of people who have come to the sensation later in life (such as in high school or early adulthood). Many first experience it in the clinical setting after being introduced to biofeedback, hypnosis, or other alternative treatments. However, others experience it organically based on the actions of others and when that happens, it can be a jarring experience.

For example, we know of a happily married man who worked with a woman whose voice triggered his ASMR. He'd never heard of the sensation before and could not understand why he seemed mesmerized by this woman. He knew he did not have romantic feelings for her, but he couldn't seem to get enough of her voice and said that she was the kind of person who could have "sold him anything" with her melodic cadence.

Unlike children who may not know what the ASMR sensation is but accept the feeling unconditionally, those who first feel it at the high school/college level or in the professional/ vocational setting say it raises feelings of confusion, especially if they have never heard of the sensation or have not experienced it in the past. In the case of the gentleman, once he learned what ASMR is and some of the triggers that caused it, he was able to discern that his colleague's voice stimulated the ASMR sensation within him.

Are you among those who may be affected by latent ASMR sensations? The following are some questions you can ask yourself to see if that's the case:

- Does a new co-worker's voice have a calming affect on you?

- Did a change in physician, hair stylist, or other professional cause you to feel more relaxed during these appointments?

- Do events that you have experienced hundreds of times in the past (such as a haircut) feel like a more relaxing experience based on the mannerisms and technique of the individual performing them?

- Have you ever confused a tingly reaction for romantic attraction?

If you answered "yes" to any of these, you might be one of those late bloomers. While we can't state this unequivocally (as everyone's situation is different), what we can tell you is that if you are among those who discovered your ASMR tingles a little later on, there is nothing wrong with you and there is nothing to be ashamed of or embarrassed by.

If you suspect that you are being triggered, try to determine how the trigger affects you on a visual, sonic, or experiential level. For example, if you discover that it is the sound of someone's voice, feel free to tell the individual (in a nice way) that her voice is very relaxing. Sometimes merely acknowledging it is enough to diffuse the trigger's impact a little. We don't know why this is, but friends have told us it works. Plus, the other person may consider it a compliment.

The following are some other suggestions:

- If it is something the other person is doing (such as a visual trigger), you may have to train yourself to avert your gaze especially at times when you cannot "enjoy the view," so to speak.

- If it is another type of sound trigger (such as snapping gum, smacking lips, tapping fingers, and so on), you may need to mask those noises by wearing earphones at those times when you need to be productive and can't be distracted by sounds that relax you.

- If you discover that you are suddenly triggered by an experience in a way you weren't in the past, feel free to indulge in the moment without being overly obvious. (In other words, try not to fall asleep.) While most people find salon/spa services fairly relaxing, consider yourself lucky if you can be triggered in a doctor's office. Not everyone can do that!

None of these suggestions are designed to discourage your ASMR. Rather, it is to help you understand it better and gain some control over what you might feel is an uncontrollable situation.

TINGLE TIP

Not every ASMR trigger is connected to a memory. Many are random combinations of sights and sounds that result in a spontaneous ASMR event (such as watching Bob Ross paint). If you have ever experienced one of these types of ASMR episodes, be aware of what is happening when the event occurs and seek out content that matches those elements. Sometimes you might be able to find the perfect combination of triggers in one video!

Finding and Expanding Your Triggers

Discovering your ASMR triggers is a trial-and-error process. Most people who connect with the concept of ASMR can recall immediately when they first felt the tingles, know what caused it, and then have a starting point to start seeking content that promotes a particular trigger. So while there is no methodology we can offer that will bring your personal triggers to the surface, we can offer the following step-by-step process as a potential aid, with the caveat that finding your triggers is a highly subjective process:

1. Identify a childhood memory that created a feeling of deep relaxation, peacefulness, and tranquility.

2. Try to remember that event as completely as possible. This goes beyond merely knowing the who, what, where, when, how, and why to include all that you felt and experienced through the five senses.

3. Determine what part of the memory had the most effect on you. Was it something you saw or heard, or was it the experience itself? (ASMR videos tend to fall into visual, auditory, and experiential categories, which we will talk more about over the next few chapters.)

4. Seek out YouTube content that focuses on what you feel is your particular trigger. Don't be discouraged if it doesn't work the first time. Try multiple ASMRtists; everyone is a little different.

5. If trying multiple videos does not work, revisit the memory to determine if there is a different trigger to try. (You may have selected the wrong one.)

While there is no formula for knowing every trigger that works for you, when you find one, it will lead to more, and from there, you can seek out content that includes the elements that are most likely to trigger your ASMR. In fact, those who transition from traditional guided meditation videos, nature soundscapes, and other content designed for relaxation to ASMR videos are often surprised to learn how their triggers can grow quickly over time.

This often occurs thanks in part to the video suggestion queue that brackets a YouTube viewer's feed. For example, we know a lot of people who might have been watching a quiet meditation video but became intrigued by the terms "ear-to-ear whisper" and "soft-spoken relaxation" enough to click on the videos and then felt amazement at the tingly effect the content had on them. Or perhaps they were reminded of how much they loved hushed voices as their teacher read a story or enjoyed the quiet soothing comments made while someone brushed their hair. The next thing they know, they are surfing YouTube for hair brushing videos, which may lead to full-on salon role-plays and more. Before you know it, they have a wide variety of ASMR content triggers to choose from!

So if you are just beginning to discover your ASMR triggers, we recommend trying a variety of videos; you never know what you might connect with if you give it a chance.

ASMR Immunity: Beating the Buzzkill

One question that comes up from time to time has to do with subject of *ASMR immunity* and whether someone can actually lose the ability to experience ASMR. While there is no real science to prove or disprove this, we don't think so. ASMR is a little like riding a bike. If you have experienced it once, you can and probably will experience it again.

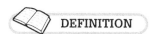 **DEFINITION**

> **ASMR immunity** is a term used to describe the sudden inability to experience the ASMR sensation when watching or listening to favorite content.

ASMR immunity occurs when an individual watches or listens to the same content over and over again until it no longer has the same effect that it once did. This happens due to a change in the way that endorphin receptors react to repeated stimuli.

Endorphin receptors have a tendency to become desensitized when exposed to the same trigger over and over in much the same way that a drug addict needs more and more of their chemical of choice in order to achieve their desired buzz. This isn't the body trying to deny you pleasure; rather, it's its way of telling you that you have become too dependent on one stimulus. This is not a bad thing.

Dr. Craig Richard, PhD, cell biologist with the University of Shenendoah, says this automatic desensitization aspect of endorphin receptors can actually help us grow and develop. He said that if, as infants, we received a pleasurable high every time we snuggled with our parents, chances are we'd never leave their side. We would never learn to walk, talk, go to school, or venture away from home. Remember that part of the ASMR experience is in the surprise. As a child, your first ASMR episodes did not happen because you were planning them. They happened when you least expected it.

If you take the time to switch up your ASMR triggers and not use the same ones all the time, you stand a better chance of avoiding this desensitization in your endorphin receptors. However, if you do end up with ASMR immunity, rest assured it is a temporary condition. "Whatever receptors are involved, they are likely to recover their sensitivity in a short period of time," he said.

Sometimes, you just need to switch things up a bit. As you become more familiar with which ASMRtists tend to trigger your tingles on a consistent basis, you can then be relatively content they usually have something on the playlist that will work, so be open to trying something new. If you are predominately triggered by visual images, try a sound trigger or a role-play.

Of course, if there is something you haven't seen done yet, you can always make a request. Be sure to be polite when contacting your favorite ASMRtists and know that not every request can be honored. Remember, they are providing you with free content that helps relax you and put you to sleep. Be grateful for the content they do provide and don't dwell on what they can't.

ASMR Videos to Help You Discover Your Triggers

If you are ready to start exploring the ASMR universe in search of triggers that might cause your brain to tingle, here are a few that will stimulate the senses and help connect you to some of the most popular memories of the past:

- **Springbok ASMR: ASMR Teacher Role-Play: Introductions to Rhetoric** (youtube. com/watch?v=IG_sYgw8rUo)

- **WhispersUnicorn: Teacher Role-Play in 3D** (youtube.com/watch?v=mgs0StdIrIU)

- **ASMR Massage Psychetruth: Wow! ASMR Hair Brushing, Head Massage with Hair Play, Soft-Spoken Whisper, 3D Binaural Relaxation** (youtube.com/ watch?v=DxBzYU5Q3n0)

- **GentleWhispering: Soft-Spoken Relaxing Hair Play** (youtube.com/ watch?v=OoNWLyNbFaY)

- **Asmrsurge: ASMR Unwrapping and Playing with Dice (Binaural)** (youtube.com/watch?v=TVRzDhBhAio)

- **JustAWhisperingGuy: ASMR Art Therapy** (youtube.com/watch?v=fFdAI7SOZno)

 KEEP IN MIND

It is impossible to know for certain how many people experience ASMR at the present time or whether the majority of people will be able to experience it in the future. While we believe that most people can derive some relaxation benefit from ASMR content with or without the tingly feeling, there may be some exceptions to the rule. Children and adults dealing with ADD/ADHD, sensory disorders, severe mental issues, and on the autism spectrum may not respond positively to ASMR content at all. Because some ASMR videos can be extremely stimulating in terms of the sounds and visual imagery, before introducing an extremely sensitive person to ASMR, be sure to clear it with your health-care professional or therapist if you think you fall into one of those categories.

The Least You Need to Know

- The majority of first-time ASMR experiences occur before the age of 10.
- Voices, hair-play, action sounds, art/writing sounds, and random touches top the list of first-time ASMR experiences.
- In order to improve your chance of tingles, look for ASMR triggers that remind you of your previous experiences.
- ASMR stimuli should connect on a multisensory level.
- ASMR immunity is a temporary condition that can be relieved by a changeup in ASMR content.

Visual Triggers:
Just One Look

They are the relaxing images you can see, hear, taste, touch, and smell. Visual montages take you on momentary mini-vacations and enable you to daydream, reflect, and reach the deepest recesses of the mind. For the ASMR community, visual triggers are a key component of the overall tingle experience. Used in concert with soft-spoken guided visualizations and sounds, they help ASMR experiencers like you focus on those actions they empathize with and find pleasurable without having to formulate the image for themselves.

In this chapter, we explore how these image-based techniques engage the senses and enable you to alter your brain wave state and relax. You also learn why you may connect with actions you do not perform and find ordinary tasks so mesmerizing, as well as how ASMRtists have mastered the art of show-and-tell.

In This Chapter

- Visual triggers: what you see and what you perceive
- How visual perception works
- What are mirror neurons?
- ASMR content that is a treat for the eyes

What Are Visual Triggers?

As you learned in Chapter 8, tingle heads come to the ASMR experience in a variety of ways. For some, that first sensation occurs in response to something that happens to them when they are very young, while other ASMR episodes are induced by events they witnessed a little later on. These stimuli are known as *visual triggers*.

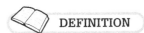 **DEFINITION**

> A **visual trigger** is an action that can lead to an ASMR episode when someone stares at it for a period of time.

A visual trigger is an image or action that is perceived by individuals through the sense of sight, resonates with them, leads to a change in brain wave state, and can ultimately result in the ASMR sensation. Visual triggers can be used alone or coupled with other practical and auditory stimuli for a multisensory ASMR experience.

Like all ASMR stimuli, visual triggers are highly subjective and do not follow specific criterion. A visual trigger may be an image or action (usually in motion) that exists in real time and operates at a speed and/or frequency that causes you to go into a trancelike state and induce an ASMR episode, or it may be mental images formulated and processed during a guided visualization exercise the brain perceives to be real. It isn't always possible to know what kind of visual trigger will work and when; the triggers are often dependent on who is using them, where the triggers are being observed, when they happen, why they occur, and under what circumstances.

Visual triggers are often methodical activities on display for everyday purposes, such as cooking and craft or art demonstrations. However, they can also be found in simple, ordinary tasks, such as gift wrapping, towel folding, or ironing. In fact, you can even get a visual trigger from watching fish swim aimlessly in an aquarium.

How Visual Triggers Work

So how do visual triggers work? You may have heard clichés like "a picture is worth a thousand words" and that "what you see is what you get." There is a lot of truth to both statements. Sight is the most influential sense you possess. Every second of every day, your brain takes mental images of everything going on around you and sends countless pieces of conscious and subconscious information to your brain.

However, visual stimulation is not limited to mental imagery. It can also include the images around you. While there are experienced tingle heads that can block everything out around them and achieve ASMR, we feel that the environment around the individual contributes to a pleasant

ASMR experience. Messy rooms, bright lights, and other visual stressors can distract from that calm, relaxing place of internal peace that can lead to ASMR.

It's no secret that visual stimulation is featured in a lot of relaxation methodologies. Yoga trainers, hypnotherapists, physicians, and clinicians often use visual imagery to help calm people's mind so they can revert to that most receptive alpha state of mind that can accept additional triggers and ultimately result in an ASMR experience.

The Perception Process

Before a visual trigger (or any other stimulus) can result in the ASMR tingles, it must go through the perceptual process. The perceptual process is the way in which human beings recognize the environmental stimuli around them and then formulate the actions that will respond to them. Although there are eight steps to the process, they happen so quickly it is impossible for you to really notice them as they occur. These steps include the following:

1. **The environmental stimulus:** This could be anything and everything in the environment that can be experienced by the five senses.

2. **The attended stimulus:** This refers to the specific object in your environment upon which your attention is focused.

3. **The image on the retina:** Light passes through the cornea and the lens of your eye in order to form an inverted image of the attended stimulus on your retina.

4. **Transduction:** This is the process of turning the image into electrical signals, which are then sent to the brain for interpretation.

5. **Neural processing:** Depending on the signal type that is received (for example, visual or auditory), the signal is then sent through a vast network of neurons to be translated.

6. **Perception:** You become consciously aware of the stimulus in your environment.

7. **Recognition:** You interpret and give meaning to what you have perceived so you can react to it.

8. **Action:** Motor action occurs in response to the stimulus. This action could be as major as running away from danger or as simple as blinking your eyes.

These last two steps are critical in the ASMR experience because as you learned in Chapter 8, in order to feel the ASMR sensation, you must be able to empathize or connect with the trigger on a cognitive level. You have to be able to stretch your sensibilities to an external event and experience it as if it is happening directly to you.

Mirror Neurons: Monkey See, Monkey Do

In order to make this connection visually, your *mirror neurons* may offer you the ability to associate the actions you perform with the actions you see and perceive. Mirror neurons are a group of cells located on either side of the brain that fire not only when you perform an action, but also when you observe someone else do it. They were discovered in the early 1990s by a team of Italian researchers studying the brain cells of macaque monkeys. They found that the neurons of a monkey's brain fired the same way both when it reached for a peanut and when it observed someone else reaching for a peanut.

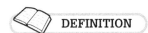 DEFINITION

Mirror neurons are brain cells that cause you to respond equally to a particular action whether you are performing that action yourself or watching it be performed by someone else.

Many scientists believe that mirror neurons not only simulate the action itself, but also the feelings and sensations that go along with it. In other words, they may help you empathize with a situation. If this theory is true (and at the present time, research is inconclusive), mirror neurons may explain why you are able to react to ASMR triggers as if you are in the middle of the action. Think about it; when you see someone play with someone's hair, you "get it," because you have some experience with that situation yourself. You are able to project your senses onto the visual in order to step into the situation and feel it what the other person is feeling.

In 2013, cognitive neuroscientist turned author Christian Jarrett evaluated research conducted in London by British scientists James Kilmer and Roger Lemon that may also be significant to the ASMR experience. After reading through 25 papers on the mirror neuron systems of monkeys, the pair concluded that the term *mirror neuron* actually hides a rather complex mix of cell types that respond very differently depending on how the visual stimulation is offered.

Jarrett noted that some of the cells only displayed mirrorlike responses when the monkey observed the action as it was being performed live, while other cells fired to actions they witnessed via video presentation. Some of the neurons were choosy, responding only to a specific type of action, while others were indiscriminate. Some were activated by sound, while other cells were reduced during observation. Some neurons were even "touch-sensitive," responding only to the sight of another monkey being touched in the same spot.

This kind of subjective triggering should sound familiar if you are a longtime tingle head or even if you are new to the ASMR experience and wonder why certain triggers induce tingles while others do not. There are so many factors that affect your ability to connect with and mirror a scenario that the only thing science can say with certainty is that the real reason is embedded deep in a complex network of brain activity.

Jarrett said although mirror neurons are an exciting and intriguing discovery, some of the hype surrounding them is speculative at best: "We're still trying to establish for sure whether they exist in humans, and how they compare to the monkey versions. As for understanding the functional significance of these cells … don't be fooled: that journey has only just begun," he said. So while these findings have provided some new information on how visual perception works, it has not been conclusively proven in humans. Still, this concept can help you understand visual triggers.

DID YOU KNOW?

At the present time, direct evidence of individual mirror neurons continues to come from studies conducted on monkeys because it is too invasive to try and study these specific cells in humans. Functional MRI tests have been conducted; however, their results where mirror neurons are concerned are difficult to interpret.

Effective ASMR Visual Triggers

In order to offer you what we feel to be some of the most popular and most effective visual ASMR triggers, it was important to determine what kinds of videos qualified for the list. Because ASMR content is intrinsically tied to YouTube, it can be argued that every video on the site (outside of audio-only tracks) constitutes as visual trigger content, but that is not the case.

Most people consider visual triggers to be those videos that feature soft-spoken guided imagery, close-range hand movements, or plenty of visual effects. Although guided visualization technically qualifies, we have eliminated image-based content that does not engage the visual sense. While we do include some video content that features up-close hand movements, we exclude those that rely too heavily on auditory triggers, such as scratching and tapping (see Chapter 10 for links to auditory trigger videos). In addition, we have also eliminated experiential videos, such as role-plays that often have a lot of special effects and plenty to see but focus more on people's ability to project themselves into the experience rather than empathize with the action being performed (see Chapter 11 for links to role-plays).

What we were left with was a satisfying category of videos that require you to focus on them visually (if only for a brief period of time), contain a pleasing array of gentle movements, and are not overpowered by vocal narratives or other sounds.

Hair Play

One of the first ASMR triggers people report typically has something to do with their hair. In many cases, it's an experiential event (which will be covered more in Chapter 11), but sometimes it occurs when watching someone else have his hair cut, styled, or brushed.

There is evidence to support the healing power of watching and/or participating in this grooming process because it takes the focus of your brain away from your own stressors and forces your thoughts onto something or someone else. Like brushing a dog or cat, folding towels, or ironing, hair play does not require a lot of thought and is something that is easily identifiable visually.

Some of our favorite hair play videos include the following:

- **asmrmassage: Hair Play Head Massage—Soft-Spoken ASMR** (youtube.com/watch?v=JtsCuz9LVr8)

- **ASMR Massage Psychetruth: Soft-Spoken Relaxing Hair Brushing and Scalp Massage** (youtube.com/watch?v=G0D9dSvrdxk)

- **TheWaterwhispers: ASMR Binaural Hair Playing and Hair Brushing** (youtube.com/watch?v=_0ZURDWrz4I)

"Draw My Life" and Whiteboard Animation Videos

If you are the kind of tingle head who could fall asleep in seconds while watching a classmate draw, "Draw My Life" or other whiteboard animation videos may be the perfect trigger for you!

Whiteboard animation is a term used to describe a recording process in which a spoken narration comes alive on whiteboard using unsophisticated comic strip–style artwork and time-lapse or stop-motion effects. These dry-erase animations have become a big trend in video presentation throughout the world and have been used by businesses, schools, organizations, and more.

Marketing experts and bloggers say what makes these videos oddly compelling is not the rudimentary artwork; it's good storytelling. People love a good story and they love to see it come to life. Also, because whiteboard animation always has a work-in-progress feel to it, people tend to want to see how it turns out, so there is a tendency to stick around until the very end. From an educational standpoint, there is also a belief that when information is offered in both a visual and auditory medium, the viewer tends to retain much more of it.

In ASMR application, the reason is a little less clear. In fact, they seem to defy logic. Unlike other videos, which tend to focus on gentle hand movements, in whiteboard animation, the hands move quickly and are juxtaposed against a soothing voice. By anyone's definition, this should be jarring, but it's not. It actually has the opposite effect.

Eli Weiner at Yes! MediaWorks says their incredibly enticing features lead many of these videos to be original, memorable, and even jaw-dropping at times: "(Normally) we associate whiteboards with the boring, everyday office environment; but we are enraptured when an artist begins to create imagery on one to go along with spoken narrative … even though it must be carefully planned, it looks spontaneous and that's part of the fun," he says. In other words, the originality of these videos could be what makes these videos visually triggering.

> **TINGLE TIP**
>
> Some of the best whiteboard animations (though not specifically geared to the ASMR community) on the web can be found at the Royal Society for the Encouragement of the Arts, Manufactures and Commerce (RSA) website: thersa.org.

Ready to try some whiteboard animation and "Draw My Life" videos? Check these out:

- **Heather Feather: Draw My Life (Soft-Spoken ASMR for Tingles, Relaxation, and Sleep)** (youtube.com/watch?v=iBKLswx1FW4)

- **Hailey WhisperingRose: ASMR: Draw My Life HD Soft Spoken** (youtube.com/watch?v=n0_h6M7h0F8)

- **JustAWhisperingGuy: Draw My Life (ASMR)** (youtube.com/watch?v=Uv3vTVd6qUI)

Aquarium Therapy

When it comes to ASMR visual triggers, aquariums are as old school as it can get. They are colorful, hypnotic, and do not require a YouTube account or even internet access. In fact, fish are so well known for having a calming and relaxing effect on individuals, this is one of the reasons so many doctor's office waiting rooms and hospital common areas have large fish tanks.

Studies have shown that just five minutes with Nemo and friends can have a positive effect on your physical and mental health. Experts believe that aquarium therapy can help with the following issues:

- Insomnia

- High blood pressure

- Stress and anxiety

- Tension

- Behavioral health problems

- Geriatric issues

- Chronic illnesses

- Soothing crying children

Plus, in addition to the visual triggers of watching fish swim around, there are the added tingles associated with the sounds of the filter and the gentle hum of the motor, giving aquariums an attractive balance in terms of trigger assortments.

While it can be fun to set up an aquarium in your own home to trigger your ASMR sensation at all times, you can also find plenty of soothing aquatic life on YouTube to help you relax or put you to sleep. The following are just a few aquarium videos:

- **TexasHighDef: Aquarium with Natural Wave Sounds** (youtube.com/watch?v=PTvBpF-bWZI)

- **Oscar Villarreal: Marine Aquarium Virtual Fish Tank** (youtube.com/watch?v=cYU_dhrmvyU)

- **Scenic Labs: BluScenes: Scenic Aquarium (Coral Reef Tank)** (youtube.com/watch?v=XjBWvP4jrOM&list=PL86D5A3C9AB3FFlb6)

TINGLE TIP

Aquariums are only one way tingle heads connect with the natural world. For some, watching the mesmerizing rise and fall of ocean waves can send them into gentle slumber. For others, it's a mountain waterfall. Feel free to explore some of these natural sounds yourself and see if they work for you.

The Special Case of Show-and-Tell Videos

Show-and-tell videos are the catchall of ASMR content. They are wildly popular segments that run the gamut in terms of presentation and the kinds of triggers that they offer. Show-and-tells can be incorporated into role-plays, are often demonstrative (such as cooking or craft how-tos), and can be composed of an assortment of interesting items an ASMRtist wants to share.

But do they qualify as visual triggers? They can, but this is largely dependent on the sensory style of the viewer, the characteristics of the featured objects, and the way in which the ASMRtist interacts with them.

As you learned in Chapter 8, individuals tend to gather information in a variety of ways, but generally speaking, they fall into one of three sensory styles where their ASMR triggers are concerned: watchers (visual learners), listeners (auditory learners), or touchers (kinesthetic learners). Watchers tend to favor visual triggers and need to actually see something on the screen. Although the item itself might make a sound if it is tapped, stroked, or adjusted in some way, the viewer must see it in order to achieve the ASMR reaction. Visual triggers are also favored by those who are predominately "touchers" because the objects featured in this type of ASMR content often contain a number of fun characteristics, including elaborate textures, luxurious fabrics, smooth surfaces, or other appealing elements. They are often the kind of thing you wish you could reach out and feel but can get a "second-hand thrill" by watching someone else do it and imagining what it would be like to explore it yourself.

These two sensory types of watching and touching are well matched with one another, especially if the viewer is primarily a watcher and the ASMRtist is primarily a toucher. The kinesthetic ASMRtist does not merely run their fingers over an item, but savors each element of it as if it were a fine meal. The gentle gestures and fluidity of movement are mesmerizing to the viewer, and even if there are sound triggers included in the video, this satisfies the need for visual stimulation.

Here are just a few show-and-tell videos geared toward the visual senses:

- **GentleWhispering: Origami Show-n-Tell "The Collection"** (youtube.com/watch?v=Tf77i2lEp1I)

- **VeniVidiVulpes: ASMR Show-and-Tell: What's in My Bag?** (youtube.com/watch?v=S16vC1lVy7A)

- **mymilkysounds: ASMR Show-and-Tell Soft Things Gentle Hand Movements** (youtube.com/watch?v=0uDo_tbq2z4)

A Study in Visual Mastery: Olivia's Kissper ASMR

While there are a number of ASMRtists who have the art of the hand movement mastered, Olivia's Kissper ASMR is among the best. Her videos are truly a treat for the eyes. Born in the Czech Republic, the ethereal blonde joined the YouTube ASMRtist community in 2013 with a hair brushing video and quickly set herself apart from the pack. No matter if she is conducting a cranial nerve examination or acupuncture treatment or taking her viewer on a guided tour of a museum, her hypnotic hands are front and center in every video she films.

Although her voice is as light as soap bubbles and ranges somewhere between a kiss and a whisper (hence the term *kissper*), her hands are the star of the show. The simplest narrative is coupled with a touch of the hair, a wiggle of a finger, or a twist of the wrist that looks as if she is conjuring a spell.

Olivia's Kissper ASMR's background in psychology, transpersonal psychology, and consciousness studies—as well as her work as an instructor of relaxation, meditation, lucid dreaming, and mindfulness methodologies—have given her unique insight into the sensory styles of her viewers. "The aim of my work is not to just pacify … but (to) really find out how we can use this pleasurable feeling of altruistic attention … to be more alive," she says on her website, feelmoreasmr.com.

In order to experience Olivia's Kissper ASMR work for yourself, check out some of these videos, which contain some of her best handwork and visual triggers:

- **Relaxing CARD Reading ASMR Soft Spoken** (youtube.com/watch?v=rm0UeEeyDGw)

- **Relax and Binaural ASMR Drawing: Whispered** (youtube.com/watch?v=ACUgFfrelOk)

- **Drawing 3D Illusion—ASMR Soft Spoken** (youtube.com/watch?v=DhQkjbwC6qo)

The Least You Need to Know

- Visual triggers must be things you perceive and empathize with.
- Mirror neurons are brain cells that enable you to recognize an action whether you perform it yourself or watch someone else perform it. These could have a bearing on people's ability to empathize.
- ASMR visual triggers are not role-plays and do not rely heavily on sound.
- ASMR show-and-tell videos can be visual triggers, depending on your sensory type and the way in which the ASMRtist reacts with featured objects.

A Symphony of Sound

They are ordinary noises that turn your brain to mush and cause your scalp to sparkle like a diamond. Whether it's something like tapping, clicking, brushing, and scratching, most people rarely notice or disregard them completely, yet they work on you like a drug.

ASMR auditory triggers are a fascinating variety of stimuli because they can come from numerous sources and can be generated in a multitude of ways. Not to mention, contrary to all that we have yet to learn about the ASMR phenomenon, there is quite a bit of solid science to back up why human beings tend to be soothed by sound.

In this chapter, we help you journey down the auditory canal to learn more about the sense of sound. We uncover different audio triggers and what it takes to help people connect to the symphony. Put your listening ears on and let's go!

In This Chapter

- How sound works
- Whispering and white noise
- Discovering tactile-acoustic triggers
- Bilateral stimulation: a side-to-side rhythm
- How binaural beats can get your head humming
- Why earphones matter to ASMR

Do You Hear What I Hear?

In order to understand how an auditory ASMR trigger affects the tingles in your head, you need to understand what sound is and how you experience it.

Sound is produced when an object releases energy in the form of a vibration and then radiates that energy in all directions from its original source. The vibrating object squeezes the surrounding molecules closer together and rarifies them by pulling them farther apart. Even though there are variations in the air pressure moving outward from the original object, the air molecules themselves stay in a fairly standard spot. As the sound wave moves forward, it reflects off any object in its path and creates more disruptions in the airspace.

There are six elements that determine how people perceive a sound wave:

- **Frequency:** The number of times per second that a sound wave cycles from positive to negative and back again. These are measured in Hertz (Hz).

- **Amplitude:** Also known as *intensity,* this refers to the strength of the sound wave—in other words, how loud or soft it is.

- **Phase:** This compares the timing between two similar sounds.

- **Direction:** This refers to knowing from where the sound originated.

- **Distance:** This is the perception of how near or far away the sound is.

- **Timbre:** Also known as *tone color,* this refers to the perceived quality of any sound's many frequencies differentiating over time.

DID YOU KNOW?

The study of sound perception is called *psychoacoustics* and is a multidisciplinary subject that concerns itself with the physical as well as the physiological ways in which sound affects people.

How You Receive Sound

Humans receive sound in two different ways: air conduction and bone conduction. Air conduction is when the sound energy moves the tympanic membrane (eardrum). In bone conduction, the sound is transmitted to the inner ear through the bones of the skull.

Have you ever wondered why your voice sounds different to you when you speak as opposed to when a recording of it is played back to you? When you speak, you perceive the sound through the bones of your skull, which conducts frequencies better than the air and results in your hearing a lower, fuller sound. However, when it is played back to you and you perceive the sound through the air, it frequently sounds higher than you expect it to. (This also explains why you hear your own head scratches at a higher frequency than others'.)

As you know, the way people typically receive and perceive sound is through the ear. The ear is a very complex organ of the body that acts not only as a sound filter, but also transfers everything it hears into information the brain can process and prioritize.

The ear is comprised of three areas that contain fragile but intricate mechanisms:

- Outer ear (the external ear and the ear/auditory canal)
- Middle ear (the ear drum and three very tiny bones)
- Inner ear (the cochlea and the auditory nerve)

When you detect a vibration, those sound waves are captured in the funnel-like structure of the external ear and directed to the eardrum by way of the auditory canal. When it reaches the eardrum, the hammer, anvil, and stirrup (the three tiny bones of the middle ear) work together in order to amplify the sound waves before transferring them to the inner ear. In the inner ear, the sound waves are transformed into electrical impulses and sent to the snail-shaped cochlea, which is filled with fluid that moves when exposed to sound waves. That movement is picked up by the sensory cells, which are responsible for sending the impulses to the brain via the auditory nerve for processing. When the impulses reach the brain (specifically the central auditory cortex), it sorts through the data, translates it into sound, and enables you to extract the sounds you need to respond to situation you are in.

It's a pretty extensive process for something that happens instantaneously. The ear receives sound at 768 mph and those waves do not slow down until they hit the auditory nerve. Even then, they remain at a whopping 200 mph, which makes sound one of the fastest senses that we have.

Hearing's Advantages Over Sight

Although hearing works in concert with sight as the primary senses, hearing has some distinct advantages over its visual counterpart. Unlike eyesight, which is forward facing, hearing is multidirectional and allows you to receive not only the information you can see but also what you can't. This helps you remain aware in your surroundings and recognize individual sounds even when there is a lot of noise. Plus, hearing is always available; you cannot temporarily cut off your sense of hearing in the same way you can eliminate your sight by closing your eyes.

In addition, hearing is critical to your ability to communicate with others. Not only does it allow you to understand the individual words that are spoken, but it enables you to discern the emotions and meaning behind them through the tone that is used to express them. For example, although the human brain processes thousands of sounds throughout the day, not surprisingly, the one it responds most to is the human voice. This is because there are special voice-sensitive regions around the primary auditory cortex that react to the emotional cues it perceives. Studies in humans, primates, and canines have determined that these areas of the brain light up more when exposed to happy sounds (laughter) as opposed to unhappy ones (screams, whines, and cries). Because of this, some scholars say the sense of hearing is the closest thing to mind reading people have.

Whispering and White Noise

Of all of the human vocalizations, the most popular ASMR trigger is the *whisper*. In fact, when we asked tingle heads about the first sounds they sought out to stimulate the ASMR sensation, whispered and softly spoken content were mentioned nearly three times more than other general sound triggers or visual stimuli. We weren't surprised. Because so many early ASMR experiences are tied to the soothing events of youth, it only makes sense that whispering is intrinsically connected to it.

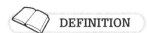

DEFINITION

A **whisper** is a pronounced means of communication that is emitted through the mouth but does not require the vocal chords to vibrate.

A whisper is a pronounced way of speaking that doesn't cause the vocal chords to vibrate. Instead, the words are hyperextended to create a certain amount of audible turbulence (hissing) on exhale that can be perceived by the listener. When someone whispers or uses a combination of whispering and soft-spoken vocalization to talk to someone, it tends to have a calming effect even if it does not produce an ASMR episode.

Whispering is a rudimentary form of sound therapy, a technique used to stimulate the pathways of the brain via frequencies that can trigger the release of hormones, such as dopamine and oxytocin. Sound therapy has been used to help listeners hear better and combat stress, fatigue, and insomnia.

Although from a clinical standpoint, sound therapy falls into the category of fringe medicine similar to biofeedback, hypnosis, and other alternative treatments, everybody knows that sound (especially music) can soothe the beast within.

According to Stephen Porges, a neuroscientist at the University of North Carolina, there is a reason for that. Apparently, there are high-frequency sounds that act like air conduction on the muscles of the middle ear and regulate those three little bones that are so precious around the eardrum. When those sounds stimulate the muscles, it can slow down the heartbeat and help you settle down.

In an interview with Radiotonic in Australia, he said the soft-spoken whispers of the ASMR community create a sensation that is not unlike the one people received when their mothers or other early caregivers used to croon lullabies to them. With the most popular ASMRtists being women, "the frequency band of female vocalization is higher, and it's that frequency which our nervous system evolved with to detect safety," he said. So the high-frequency, softly spoken ASMR vocalization content creates the feeling that everything is going to be alright.

While whispering or soft-spoken language is usually the first and one of the most common forms of sound therapy for tingle heads, it's far from the only one. There are a number of ways that sounds that can have a soothing effect on people, many of which fall into the category of *white noise.*

Similar to the idea of white light being created from every color within the spectrum, white noise is a conglomeration of all sound frequencies that result in a kind of nothingness. The resulting pitchless sound can then be used to mask all other individual sounds around it and give listeners something upon which to concentrate.

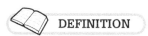

DEFINITION

White noise is a collection of sound vibrations that contain all known frequencies and result in a pitchless nothingness, which is used to mask other sounds.

Though it may sound absurd to mask noise with more noise, it's really not when you stop to think about it. Have you ever lived or worked near a construction zone and become so distracted by the resulting noise that you turned on the TV or some music to drown out the noise from beyond? That is the perfect example of how you can use white noise to build a better environment.

The broad category of white noise can include any number of background noises that can be used to help people sleep, meditate, or focus on a specific task. For example, there are a number of individuals who are steadfast in their need to have a ceiling fan running above them in order to sleep at night. There are also some who can't walk into a room or work without the sound of the television or radio in the background (even if they aren't watching it), and still others who are simply soothed by environmental noises found on white noise machines, recordings, and CDs that give them a sense they are far from their everyday lives.

Some of the most popular white noise sounds include the following:

- Ocean waves and other water sounds (for example, a babbling brook, waterfalls, and rain)

- Nature sounds (for example, birds, crickets, wind through the trees, and thunder)

- A fan or small motor sounds

- Music, especially classical, folk, or other gentle compositions

- The drone of home shopping channels, often used because it helps individuals feel less alone

A whisper is an example of white noise because it is created by turbulent airflow that emits different pitches simultaneously. However, because it lacks intensity and penetration and cannot be heard from far away, it tends to blend into other environmental sounds.

Are you interested in the sound therapy of whispering and white noise? The following videos can get you started:

- **GentleWhispering: Mirror Relaxation Whisper Video** (youtube.com/watch?v=x7ca_Msca2Q)

- **WhispersForListeners: Whisper #1 Relaxation/Stress Reduction Guided Meditation/Hypnosis** (youtube.com/watch?v=sNNU60HyYXY)

- **WhisperingLife: Whisper 77** (youtube.com/watch?v=4rMLPxQOYes)

- **Whisper Crystal: Whisper Peaceful Sleep Relaxation** (youtube.com/watch?v=DVXQpnHL74o)

- **Relaxing White Noise: Waterfall—Nature's Best White Noise for Relaxation and Sleep** (youtube.com/watch?v=1KAE_JJx0-I)

- **Ultimate Relax Club: 10 Hours Rain and Thunder Healing Ambient Sounds for Deep Sleeping Meditation Relaxation Spa** (youtube.com/watch?v=Sv0LwXYAVVg)

- **Outstanding Videos: Relaxing Three-Hour Video of a Tropical Beach with Blue Skies, White Sands, and Palm Trees** (youtube.com/watch?v=qREKP9oijWI)

Tactile-Acoustic Triggers

ASMR auditory content is about more than whispering and white noise. In fact, it contains a vast library of ordinary, everyday sounds that have become the most addicting thing since caffeine in recent years. Why is that, and what is it about scratching fabric, tapping on a cell phone, and crinkling candy wrappers that is so euphoric?

It is a question with several possible answers. The easiest is that the *tactile-acoustic trigger* is connected to a specific event in people's lives and when they hear it, it conjures memories of that experience. A quick and efficient tapping sound may remind you of the way your teacher's heels clicked against the classroom floor. The scratch of upholstery fabric may remind you of the sofa your grandmother used to have and how you used to do the same thing in order to call her cat. Whatever the trigger may be, when you hear it, you are transported back to that time and place and, if it is a pleasant memory, it gives you an extra shot of oxytocin or dopamine and a tingly sensation that you want to experience again and again.

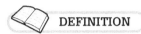 **DEFINITION**

> A **tactile-acoustic trigger** is a touch-based sensation that results in a pleasurable sound (for example, popping bubble wrap, tapping fingers, clicking blocks together, shuffling cards, and so on).

Although a lot of people who do not experience ASMR may think of these triggers as odd, they are not as strange as you might think. Individuals use various tactile acoustic triggers to self-soothe at times when they are most anxious. You've probably seen this kind of behavior if you know someone on the autism spectrum. It is a protective response that results in an individual needing to "self-stimulate" in order to regain control over their body and relieve anxiety. However, it's fairly common in nonautistic people as well. You probably know many people who twirl their hair, tap their foot, or whistle absentmindedly. The difference between autism spectrum self-stimulation and self-stimulation in people without autism is that the latter have more control over those stimulations and seem to have a better grasp on what is acceptable to do in public.

Although the sound itself may seem fairly ordinary, like visual triggers, they are often presented in deliberate ways. There is care taken to make sure that every sound is audible, is a little slower, and is as effective as it can be. Merely wadding a piece of paper will have no effect on someone, but if it's done slowly and gently, it may hit the right frequency in someone's brain to help the person achieve ASMR.

Some of the most popular ASMR tactile-acoustic triggers include the following:

- **Tapping:** Glass, metal, wood, and plastic objects are the most popular tapping videos.

- **Scratching:** Fabric tends to be the most popular, but any textured item can make a satisfying scratching sound.

- **Brushing:** This trigger is usually performed directly on the microphone itself and is often unseen by the viewer.

- **Picking:** This is another trigger that is often performed gently on the microphone itself, though it can be done on an object that has a unique texture.

- **Crinkling:** Plastic candy wrappers, aluminum foil, and paper are the most popular crinkles.

- **Nonenvironmental water sounds:** This refers to pouring, swishing, bubbling, dripping, and so on.

- **Clicking:** Video game controller sounds as well as the sound of handling plastic and wood blocks are among fan favorites.

ASMR "sound slices" (the term for a collection of auditory sounds) include a number of these kinds of triggers within a single segment. Some of our favorites include the following:

- **SonographicSoothe: Tingle Fairy Ear Cleaning (ASMR Sounds)** (youtube.com/watch?v=OBZiuq3iVjw)

- **Heather Feather: ASMR Binaural Sound Slice: Ear Exam/Hearing Test (Tuning Fork, Ear Covering, Latex Gloves)** (youtube.com/watch?v=0KHkgqGeSFU)

- **ThatASMRChick: ASMR Various Plastic Box Sounds + Crinkling/Tapping/ Scratching (No Talking)** (youtube.com/watch?v=CGlo6_hOItk)

- **TheWaterwhispers: 3 Different Triggers for Sleep—ASMR Whispering** (youtube.com/watch?v=2v855i_6YFc)

Bilateral Stimulation

Another audio technique that many ASMRtists employ in order to help their fans get the most out of their listening experience is *bilateral stimulation*. Bilateral stimulation is a process in which someone uses visual, auditory, or tactile stimuli in a rhythmic side-to-side pattern. Passing a beanbag from one hand to the other is an example of bilateral stimulation.

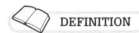

> **DEFINITION**
>
> **Bilateral stimulation** is a process in which someone uses visual auditory or tactile stimuli in a side-to-side pattern for therapeutic purposes.

While they cannot employ tactile methods of bilateral stimulation in ASMR videos without viewers consciously participating, content creators often move their hands from side to side in order to have viewers follow their movements with their eyes and use binaural microphones to trigger one ear and then the other. (This is another reason why earphones are important to the ASMR experience, which we'll get into more later in this chapter.)

Bilateral stimulation has been shown to do the following:

- Result in relaxation and decreased physiological excitement

- Increase your ability to open your mind and become less focused on a particular stressor

- Create a sense of distance between you and whatever problems you are having so you are most likely to relax and get some rest

- Relieve you of your worries for the present time

The following are some bilateral stimulation videos you can check out:

- **Jorge Henderson Collazo: Bilateral Stimulation (Listen with Headphones)** (youtube.com/watch?v=_k2HMSIxK0k)

- **MusicSedona: EMDR Music Therapy/EMDR Therapy for Posttraumatic Stress Disorder (PTSD) Official** (youtube.com/watch?v=8dQXcnkHs6o)

- **jerrybacik: EMDR Plus Bilateral Sound for Racing Thoughts** (youtube.com/watch?v=OVi7yX9X35A)

 KEEP IN MIND

Although bilateral stimulation is a very safe and relaxing methodology for most tingle heads, because it is a direct sensory stimulation of the nervous system, there are some conditions for which it is not appropriate for ASMR use. These conditions—such brain injuries, migraine sufferers, complex PTSD, and dissociative identity disorder—often result in hypersensitivity to sensory stimuli. Therefore, it is critical if you suffer from any of these conditions to consult with your personal health-care physician before using any bilateral ASMR content.

Neuroacoustics

In Chapter 6, you discovered that sound is at the core of the human existence. Not only is it the only sense you use prior to birth and the sense responsible for your first memories, but we also know that human beings have been using it for thousands of years to reach deeper states of consciousness and increased awareness and as a tool for healing the body, heart, mind, and spirit. It only stands to reason that it can still be used today.

Leading the way in this field of study for the past 35 years is Jeffrey Thompson, DC, founder of the Center for Neuroacoustic Research in Carlsbad, California. Since 1980, Dr. Thompson has been on the cutting edge of neuroacoustics and the various therapeutic applications of sound. His research has led to the development of specific practices that can be used to alter one's brain wave patterns, change sympathetic and parasympathetic balance, and coordinate the activity between the two hemispheres of the brain. He has also used these methods in a number of health-related areas, including stress reduction, behavioral health, cardiovascular disease prevention, depression, and more.

Unlike traditional music therapy, which is about the individual's personal expression, Thompson said that his work involves the direct application of precise sound combinations that are specific to the individual to encourage physiological responses. "Using this technology as a daily tool for mind-body integration and stress reduction can have many positive benefits," he noted on his website.

One of the techniques Thompson specializes in is brain wave entertainment. Brain wave entertainment or "binaural beats" is a relaxation practice in which an auditory brain stem response results when two different impulses (that are not quite in tune with one another) are played in opposite ears at the same time. When the two signals come together, it produces a third sensation in the brain and, as the two wax and wane, it creates a wavy sound that is perceived as a fluctuating rhythm between the other two pulses.

This process is known to create a kind of hemisphere synchronicity in the mind and is affiliated with the brain's "a-ha moment," which typically doesn't last too long. This technique prolongs the process and has been shown to help people alleviate pain and improve cognitive function. Plus, some people say that a binaural beat of 4 cycles per second can result in the feeling of an out-of-body experience.

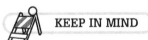 **KEEP IN MIND**

Some people have claimed that binaural beats are "digital drugs" and can simulate the effects of recreational stimulants. This has not been proven, nor have claims that they help individuals stop smoking, lose weight, or improve athletic performance.

Studies show that binaural beats have a relaxing effect and can be used to change your brain wave state in order to stimulate focus and attention as necessary. They have also been known to result in the ASMR sensation just by listening to them, which is why they have been incorporated into ASMR YouTube content.

Here are a few links to give you an example of how they work:

- **Olivia's Kissper ASMR: Futuristic Tingles! Binaural ASMR Exam and Transpersonal Healing Role-Play with Binaural Beats** (youtube.com/watch?v=PGLMHwpeghY)

- **asmrnovastar: ASMR (HD) Whisper Travel into Space—Part 1: Binaural Beats, Panning, and Tapping** (youtube.com/watch?v=mIjIzz9z_3w)

- **psyphi70: Binaural Beats—Alpha to Theta—Deepening Waves 3D Sound—ASMR** (youtube.com/watch?v=_ho1obOFjNs)

Using Earphones to Listen to ASMR

If you were to ask 100 ASMR experiencers about how they listen to ASMR content, you would probably get 100 different opinions. There is a general consensus that if you can't experience the ASMR sensation without earphones, it is unlikely the addition of them will improve your chances. However, if you can achieve ASMR without earphones (or with a cheap pair found in a clearance bin), it is a safe bet they will only add to your ASMR experience.

Some tingle heads say that ear buds are the best for ASMR because they send the trigger straight into your ear. Still, others prefer the more traditional over-the-head options. While there is a wealth of options on the market, the following are just some of the ones that come highly recommended by ASMR experiencers:

- **Beats by Dr. Dre ($299):** A little pricey and hotly debated online, these are favorites among those who want an enhanced ASMR experience.

- **Bose Quiet Comfort ($299):** These ear bud–style headphones are recommended for mobile devices. Like Beats, the Bose name is one tingle heads either love or hate.

- **Beyerdynamic DT 770 PRO, 80 ohms ($270):** This closed-back model is good for outside sound noise reduction.

- **Sennheiser HD 598 headphones ($181):** These headphones are particularly good for high-quality, binaural sounds.

- **Sennheiser ear buds ($39.99):** This is a proven name in headphones with a style some tingle heads swear by.

- **Sony ZX series ($17.99):** These are good-quality, over-the-head earphones for a reasonable price.

Keep in mind, however, that earphone and ear bud technology is always evolving and changing. Models that we recommend today may not be top-of-the-line or readily available a year from now. When shopping for your perfect pair, be sure to seek out those devices that offer you a good fit and are comfortable enough to allow the ASMR content go right into your brain.

The Least You Need to Know

- The sense of sound has distinct advantages over eyes, such as being multidirectional and helping you understand words and the emotion behind them.
- Whispers and white noise are two of the most popular ASMR sound triggers.
- Tactile-acoustic triggers are made up of ordinary objects that make sounds that are pleasurable.
- Brain wave entertainment is a part of neuroacoustics that can coordinate the sides of the brain and help influence conscious state.
- Earphones can enhance the ASMR experience.

The Intimacy of ASMR Role-Play

It begins with a warm, welcoming greeting by a soft-spoken individual who smiles gently and explains the event that is about to occur. No matter what it is, there is nothing to fear and no one can harm you. In fact, a few minutes into the session, you may be fast asleep. That's all right; your host won't mind. Actually, that might even be the goal.

Welcome to ASMR role-play, a facet of ASMR content that engages viewers on a personal level and brings them into the experience. Unlike segments in which the action is merely described or demonstrated for you, in the ASMR role-play, you are actually part of the show.

In this chapter, we explore what makes the ASMR role-play so special; the psychology behind its success; and why so many people can't get enough of virtual spas, cranial nerve exams, and ASMR makeup artists.

In This Chapter

- ASMR role-play: an interactive experience
- Personalized attention in an impersonal world
- How ASMR videos simulate the sights and sounds of everyday life
- The most common ASMR role-play scenarios

A Rundown of Role-Play

One of the most popular types of ASMR content on YouTube, *role-play* is an artificial scene designed to simulate a relaxing experience through remote sensory stimulation. During this interactive segment, the ASMRtist leads the viewer (or listener) through a predetermined process that has a semidefinite storyline. In many cases, the content creator may assume a character-like persona and act out the part with dialogue, sounds, and props appropriate to the presentation.

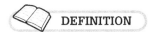
DEFINITION

A **role-play** is an artificial scenario designed to re-create a real or imagined situation.

Role-play is significantly different than traditional show-and-tells, gentle narratives, and sounds-only segments. In an ASMR role-play, the action is not merely performed for you, it's performed *on* you, as if you are actually in the room with the ASMRtist as a secondary character in the play. In ASMR, the suggestion of touch and its accompanying sound is something that sets the practice apart from other relaxation methodologies that focus on visualization and the individual's imagination. Touch is the language of compassion and has been known to have a certain amount of healing power. By supplying someone with an extra bit of sensory stimulation, it can help you connect more to the presentation, give you additional triggers, and enable you to relax more quickly.

The settings for ASMR role-plays are wide and varied. Many of the early (and current) ASMR role-play videos centered on everyday experiences that most people have some familiarity with, as well as elaborate fantasies with a number of computer-generated special effects. While they run the gamut in terms of backdrop, at the heart of every role-play is the personal attention given to the viewer through a caring and thoughtful but nonsexual experience.

The Personal Connection Provided by Role-Plays

While it's no secret that everyone needs a hug or a pat on the back from time to time, there is a lot of speculation as to why role-play content is so favored throughout the ASMR community. One persistent theory suggests the personal care and attention displayed in these videos is similar to that of the "grooming" practices found in other primate groups (such as chimpanzees, baboons, and apes). Another popular theory is that the need for artificial interaction reflects a deep need for connection in an increasingly isolated world.

The truth probably lies somewhere in the middle. There is no question that human beings have an intrinsic need for interpersonal interaction; it's no secret that some ASMR role-plays are used to help reconnect people to those events of the past they found soothing, such as their mother caring for them when they were sick, brushing their hair, or reading them a story. However, it is also true that despite modern technology enabling people to be more connected than ever, the population as a whole has been lulled into a false sense of friendship and camaraderie that belies the fact they are living increasingly lonely lives. As a result, the ASMR role-play may be, ironically, salvaging a sense of human intimacy in the digital age.

So in addition to the tingly goodness associated with whispers or soft-spoken speech, role-plays provide connection and intimacy for viewers who need a little TLC or to take a little break from the stressors in their lives. It allows them to feel better knowing that someone, even if only on a virtual level, understands their stress and is willing to comfort them throughout their ordeal. ASMRtists, in turn, take this responsibility very seriously and give their viewers a shoulder to cry on, so to speak.

For example, one of the most basic role-play segments is the caring friend role-play. In it, the ASMRtist portrays a friend who has come to spend the day with you, take care of you if you are sick, or snap you out of doldrums to get ready for a night on the town. During this visit, the conversation will not be interrupted by texts and there are no phone calls to return. You have the content creator's full attention and you can rest assured you will receive plenty of positive affirmations during this time.

Though there are few sounds other than the content creator's voice, the caring friend role-play offers a kind of bedside manner that few physicians can replicate. There is no demand on you other than to sit back and receive the love and support being sent through the screen; however, you are given the opportunity to reciprocate that love and caring via comments to the ASMRtist.

TINGLE TIP

If you'd like to see some caring friend role-plays, some of our favorites are Tony Bomboni's role-play for taking care of a sick friend (youtube.com/watch?v=HgnEKWPANDI), amalzd's soft-spoken caring friend role-play (youtube.com/watch?v=K9WpB3YPsOI), and JustAWhisperingGuy's caring friend role-play for panic attacks (youtube.com/watch?v=f9YGDKtsTC4).

Salon Service Role-Plays

When we asked tingle heads what role-plays had the biggest triggering effect on them, salon service role-plays was one of the top ones mentioned.

Hair play is one of the first ASMR memories many tingle heads can recall from an early age and one of the few triggers they experience regularly throughout their lives. For instance, as a child, you may easily remember a warm, fuzzy feeling that occurred when you were still reliant on others for your daily grooming habits. You might have felt a brush, comb, or fingers rake along your scalp and known the tingles would not be far behind. Later in life, the feeling might have been relegated to slumber parties and sleepovers, when an ambitious friend wanted to try out a new 'do and eventually ebbed to those once-a-month salon visits when you placed your hair in someone else's hands not only to look and feel better but in hopes of recapturing a familiar feeling from days gone by: the ASMR sensation.

There are two main reasons why the salon service role-play is so popular with ASMR experiencers. First of all, it is one of the most familiar. Who hasn't had their hair shampooed, cut, and styled at some point in their lives? Because people have experience with the sights, sounds, and sensations associated with a salon visit, it makes it much easier to superimpose themselves onto the scene.

The second reason is a bit more psychological. While a salon visit is without a doubt a relaxing and calming experience, there is something very unique about the hairdresser-client relationship. As a trained professional, a hairdresser is not only hired to help people alter their physical appearance. Over time, he becomes privy not only to the client's hair care preferences, but also to that person's innermost opinions, thoughts, and feelings. The only other relationship that can compare to it is the one between a doctor/therapist and their patient.

 DID YOU KNOW?

ASMR experiencers say their favorite part of the salon role-play is the scalp massage because it simulates the stimulation of the nerves and blood vessels around the head while calming tension at the same time.

Why is this, and how is this replicated in an ASMR video? In both situations, there is an incredible amount of trust placed in the professional. Clients trust their hairdressers not to take too much off the top or dye their hair a wild shade, while tingle heads count on ASMRtists to keep things low key and soothing and to not make a radical departure from what is commonly associated from the salon experience. There is also something about the positioning and gaze of the professional that has a bearing on the person "in the chair." Both a stylist and an ASMRtist tend to have a gentle gaze and intense focus on the job at hand, but neither of is looking at the person directly. In a salon, the stylist addresses the person through the reflection in the mirror, while in an ASMR role-play, the screen provides a similar barrier. This makes for a less invasive experience.

Plus, both events take place in an affirming, nonjudgmental atmosphere. A stylist's job is not to tear clients down; it is to lift them up and help them feel good about themselves. An ASMRtist does the same thing in his role-plays. The ASMRtist offers appropriate compliments, validates the viewer's choices, and does not criticize the viewer's preferences. His job is not to pressure viewers into changing their lives or to eliminate negative behavior, but rather to offer a supportive setting in which viewers can relax and enjoy some much-needed personal time.

Salon role-plays are not only limited to haircuts and highlights; you can also find ones that include a wide variety of day spa services as well, such as manicures, pedicures, massage therapy, and makeup artistry. The following are a few of our favorites:

- **GentleWhispering: Steamy Dreamy Spatenious ASMR** (youtube.com/ watch?v=3h4inWX8NtA)

- **ASMR Massage Psychetruth: Binaural ASMR Spa #2, Manicure and Hand Massage** (youtube.com/watch?v=SYQq3wAMVbw)

- **chelseamorganwhispers: ASMR Role-Play Makeup Application** (youtube.com/ watch?v=q_FtaGoOspU)

- **MassageASMR: ASMR Role-Play Relaxation Session with an ASMR Artist 6— Haircut and Head Massage** (youtube.com/watch?v=Rybj4C4G8uw)

DID YOU KNOW?

The makeover is second only to hair services when it comes to favorite ASMR role-plays that focus on aesthetics. In these, ASMRtists "talk" a person through a traditional makeover by showing someone products and then pretending to apply them. There are usually a lot of "container sounds" (such as opening bottles and jars) and a lot of brushing on the microphone to give the illusion of application.

Medical Role-Plays

Medical examination role-plays are an interesting branch of the ASMR universe. Even though they rank as the number-one ASMR role-play throughout the online tingle community, they are the scenarios least likely to be connected to early, real-life ASMR experiences. (The exception to this is a head lice check, but that does not count, as a licensed professional does not always conduct it.)

It's not surprising when you stop and think about it. Your earliest memories of doctor's visits are likely associated with the unpleasantness of immunizations followed by the fear that routine checkups could turn into fatal diagnoses when you are older. So why are so many tingle heads drawn to those situations that lack positive associations in real life?

Mainly because they know nothing can go wrong. In an ASMR medical exam, there is no danger of being diagnosed with cancer, receiving an astronomical bill, or being referred to a specialist for further testing. When the possible negativity affiliated with a real-life scenario is removed, all that's left are the comforting aspects of the situation: the caring and sympathetic personal attention, gentle gazes, and the implication of interpersonal interaction.

According to Danielle Orfi of the *New York Times*, there is something inherently comforting about the physical exam, especially when people know that nothing is seriously wrong. In her article "Not on the Doctor's Checklist, but Touch Matters," she notes that like salon services, the doctor-patient exchange is fundamentally different than any other relationship in individuals' lives because it includes the laying on of hands, and when people come to the doctor, they expect a physical connection. "A doctor's visit is not a doctor's visit until a stethoscope has probed the inner rhythms of the heart, and a set of medical hands has palpated the belly," she wrote.

Another reason tingle heads gravitate to the medical exam is because it has traditional relaxation methodologies built into its very core, even though many people do not realize it. Think about it: If someone comes to you running, panting and panicking, what is the first thing you tell the person to do? Take a deep breath. When you are nervous before speaking in public or going on stage, what do you do to relax the nerves? You take a deep breath. How do you begin exercise sessions? By taking some deep breaths to get the oxygen flowing. How do you start to meditate? Your clear your mind and concentrate on your breathing. How do hypnotists begin to get you into that alpha state of mind? They encourage you to concentrate on your breath. And what does a doctor do (in general) when he walks into the room? That's right. He gets his stethoscope, listens to your heart and lungs, and tells you to take a deep breath.

 TINGLE TIP

All tingle heads have practical experience with medical exams, making them one of the easiest role-plays on which to superimpose the senses. When an image is re-created faithfully in the mind, ASMR experiencers say that they can trick their brains into feeling the elements of the exam even though no one is physically touching them.

Which one of those situations is the easiest to imagine and concentrate on? The first few aren't very calming, so you can eliminate them. And if you are like us, the meditation example of clearing your head or merely focusing on your breath can seem rather daunting. Unlike those examples, the final example with the doctor is both calming and familiar, making it the easiest image to re-create mentally.

ASMR medical role-plays are traditionally noninvasive or semi-invasive exams that typically include basic intake questions, a brief explanation of what is about to occur, the exam itself, and then your discharge instructions. (Don't worry, we have a feeling you will get a clean bill of health!) Some of the most popular medical exams include cranial nerve exams (an ASMR community favorite), ear cleanings, eye exams, general check-ups, dental visits, physical/occupational therapy consultations, and hypnosis/therapy sessions.

Because the medical based role-play is the most popular ASMR category, there are numerous videos to choose from. However, in order to get you started, the following are a few we like that will help you sit back, relax, and enjoy the tingly goodness to follow:

- **Heather Feather: Binaural (3D) Cranial Nerve Exam for Tingles, Relaxation, and Sleep** (youtube.com/watch?v=BJ8EBBTEb0o)

- **TranquilLily ASMR: ASMR Binaural Ear Cleaning Role-Play—Soft Spoken and Whisper, Close Ear Sounds** (youtube.com/watch?v=3i-16fMipYw)

- **The Waterwhispers: Eye Checkup Optometrist Role-Play—Testing Your Eyes ASMR** (youtube.com/watch?v=gGicUObGJ2Y)

- **yawnblahblahblah: ASMR Yearly Physical Exam Role-Play** (youtube.com/watch?v=rycNQoMxM2w)

- **Fairy Char ASMR: ASMR Binaural Dental Visit Role-Play and Carrying You Home** (youtube.com/watch?v=0dkomdBofYA)

- **ASMRrequests: Physical Therapist Role-Play—Binaural ASMR—Soft Spoken, Personal Attention, Ear to Ear** (youtube.com/watch?v=VsZMFrup_lc)

- **TheOneLilium: A Relaxing Visit to the Therapist ASMR** (youtube.com/watch?v=5cgloRtlHZ8)

Other Service-Based Role-Plays

In addition to providing fake haircuts, highlights, and medical exams to their cadre of clients, content creators are constantly on the lookout for situations that will lend themselves well to the ASMR experience. Some of these include tutorial sessions, tarot card readings, suit fittings, interior design consultation, shop visits, and more.

Although they run the gamut in terms of setting, dialogue, and corresponding sound assortments, at their core, they are all service-based scenarios in which the ASMRtist consults with viewers on a particular issue or problem, presents them with appropriate options, and ultimately affirms their choices. What makes these role-plays unique is the fact that viewers can select the ones that might trigger them based on experience and personal preference. Let's look at some of the more common service-based role-plays and see if any of these sound like appealing options to you:

ASMR tutoring session or classroom role-play: This is one that has definite significance for a lot of tingle heads. As you learned in Chapter 8, many people say their first ASMR experience happened in the classroom, whether it was a teacher's voice or other classroom noise that triggered them. In traditional classroom videos, there is not a lot of personal interaction between the teacher and you, the student. Rather, there are plenty of perfunctory movements, including the sound of a pointer on a map, soft chalk on the blackboard, page turning, or ones associated with flash cards as you are drilled on math facts or vocabulary.

ASMR suit fitting role-play: This is a role-play that includes a lot of interaction between the tailor and you, the client. In this situation, the ASMRtist portrays a custom suit maker who must measure you for a new outfit. The ASMRtist will show you many of the tools of the trade before coming close to take a variety of measurements and making adjustments concerning overall fit. He may also show you a variety of fabrics from which you can choose your new clothes.

> **TINGLE TIP**
>
> If you are not a man or someone who can be tingled by the idea of a suit fitting, there are variations on this role-play that involve bridal gowns.

ASMR fortune-teller role-play: Like the tutoring session, there is no implied physical connection between the ASMRtist and the viewer, but you can count on a lot of ethereal gestures, intense gazes, and affected speech to be part of this role-play. An ASMRtist may gaze into a crystal ball, chart your horoscope, or conduct a full tarot reading to offer you insight into the status of your life and to warn you of what's to come. This role-play is a lot of fun, but please keep in mind that any occultlike role-play does not necessarily reflect a personal interest or belief in the supernatural and that any fortune, advice, or horoscope reading is intended for entertainment and tingle purposes only.

Consultation role-play: This is primarily demonstrative and centers on a consultation with some kind of service provider such as a shop clerk, interior designer, or fashion consultant. These role-plays are similar to the traditional show-and-tells mentioned in Chapter 9 but are set against the backdrop of some kind of storyline. (They are also one of the simplest role-plays to create. See Chapter 14 for more on how to make this type of role-play.)

If you are ready to get out of the doctor's office and day spa and into one of these other types of role-plays, we suggest the following service-based role-plays that will give you an idea of the ASMR trigger library that is available online:

- **WhispersRedASMR: Childhood ASMR Triggers #3 Teacher's Stories School Storytime Role-Play** (youtube.com/watch?v=DlQk0jaX2dk)

- **QueenOfSerene: 3D Sound—Gentleman's Suit Fitting** (youtube.com/watch?v=iohCbBoqYNc)

- **Olivia's Kissper ASMR: Relaxing Card Reading ASMR Soft Spoken** (youtube.com/watch?v=rm0UeEeyDGw)

Fantastic Fantasies: Redefining Traditional Role-Plays

Whenever a certain kind of role-play becomes popular, it seems as though every ASMRtist offers their variation on it. This is actually quite common, especially in medical exams, salon services, or tutorials. Because all of these have traditional formats and most people are familiar with them, there is not a lot of room for deviation.

Unfortunately, this leads to role-play burnout, a nonofficial condition that ASMRtists describe as trying to make something new out of the tried and true. While viewers may want more ear examinations or cranial nerve evaluations, ASMRtists can only reinvent the wheel so many times before becoming bored. To combat that, they begin to look at the elements of their most popular videos and discover how they can use them in new ways to make the ideas fresh and interesting to viewers. This has led to the creation of role-plays with a sci-fi or fantasy twist.

Taking ASMR to the Next Level

As ASMR content has changed over the past few years, so, too, have the technologies that are being used to create it. Once upon a time, ASMR videos were made almost exclusively with point-and-shoot camera applications on cell phones and other mobile devices. Today, however, ASMRtists are going high tech and purchasing top-of-the-line cameras and binaural microphones and incorporating any number of special effects. Not only has this enabled them to build a better mousetrap, so to speak, it has allowed them to completely transform the role-play as people know it.

Naturally, this has been embraced by some and eschewed by others, but that is all part of the subjectivity of the medium. Some feel that layered sounds, CGI graphics, and fanciful storylines offer tingle heads something new to trigger the senses, while others find all of the bells and whistles too stimulating and subscribe to a "less-is-more" mentality. While we are not here to offer commentary on which type of role-play is better than the other, we can say that when these impressive effects are used in concert with other aspects of ASMR content, the result is truly a treat!

Venturing into Fantasy: Ally "ASMRrequests"

Leading the way with these sci-fi and fantasy-based films is Ally "ASMRrequests." Ally "ASMRrequests" is a virtual reality enthusiast and sci-fi buff who first incorporated the type of special effects she would later become known for in her choose-your-own-adventure spa tour video (see the end of this chapter for the link to it).

The episode was her answer to the many requests she had to create a day spa video similar to all of the other ones she had seen on YouTube. Inspired to do something that had not been done before and having an affinity for the "choose your own adventure" books of her childhood, she decided to resurrect the medium ASMR style. The 11-minute video is a short introduction to the Lumous Day Spa, which features a seamless green screen background, fantastic sound quality, and three embedded links at the end to take viewers to the next stop on the tour. It was an impressive effort to say the least, and with nearly 300,000 views, it marked a new day for ASMR content creation.

TINGLE TIP

If you choose to screen the spa tour video from Ally "ASMRrequests" on a mobile device, follow the links in the description box to see other rooms on the tour. Each one has its own triggers, and you don't want to miss out on any of them!

Two months later, Ally "ASMRrequests" followed that initial breakthrough day spa video with a video on space travel (a link to this is at the end of the chapter). This video not only eclipsed its predecessor with over 1.5 million views but also included even more elaborate special effects. For example, she begins by tapping on a holographic screen and highlighting a travel package to a remote planet called Glesa 581G. When the unseen viewer agrees to the price, she begins booking the trip, conducting a background check (for the unrestricted provinces of the planet), and making sure that the viewer's "nano biology" is up to date.

Andy Williams, writer for the UK online magazine *Metro*, called it the "*Avatar* of ASMR role-play" and quite the accomplishment for someone who produced the whole thing from her living room. However, special effects aside, it's actually a fairly traditional ASMR video. Ally "ASMRrequests" has managed to offer a viewer personalized attention against a sci-fi backdrop and include a wide variety of triggers from several service-based role-plays (including the medical exam) without worrying whether anyone will claim it's inauthentic.

Plus, by creating content that does not blur the line between her relationships with her audience, she is able to give her viewers the triggers they want without subjecting herself to the more provocative elements of the ASMR community (such as girlfriend role-plays).

Sci-Fi/Fantasy Role-Play Videos

Ready to transform the way you look at ASMR role-plays? Check out these fantastic videos that take the role-play to the next level—and take you on an adventure you cannot possibly imagine!

- **ASMRrequests: ASMR Spa Tour—Choose Your Own Adventure** (youtube.com/watch?v=k9HXt6YKH_I)

- **ASMRrequests: Departure Ep. 1: Departure (or "Space Travel Agent")—ASMR Sci-Fi Series** (youtube.com/watch?v=oapgiZc5i-g&list=UUX70sfic86MKcid2n0mmmqg&index=100)

- **Heather Feather: Candy Queen ASMR Role-Play for Relaxation** (youtube.com/watch?v=s_L2LKtOXHY)

- **Tony Bomboni (ASMRer): ASMR Virtual Hotel Tour** (youtube.com/watch?v=zqUcyCpaAWY)

The Least You Need to Know

- In addition to offering tingle triggers, ASMR role-plays simulate personalized attention, which helps people feel less lonely and more connected.

- The two most popular types of ASMR role-plays are salon services and medical exams.

- Service-based videos are a step up from traditional show-and-tell episodes and allow viewers to select the ones that might trigger them based on experience and personal preference.

- ASMRtists such as Ally "ASMRrequests" are working to take role-play to the next level with futuristic sci-fi and fantasy without losing the traditional ASMR role-play components.

PART

4

Applying ASMR

ASMR episodes are random events that can be brought about by any number of influences around people. At the heart of it all, though, is someone taking the time to offer that personal care and attention others just can't get everywhere.

When it comes to on-demand events, ASMRtists are the masters of the grand illusion. In addition to using a variety of props and everyday items to re-create familiar sounds and experiences, they also research their role-plays carefully, painstakingly pen their scripts, and spend hours rendering footage until they have a seamless video to share with their viewers.

If you have ever thought of developing your own ASMR technique, this is the part for you. You learn about "everyday" ASMR you can use to help others, as well as how to create the YouTube footage everyone is talking about.

CHAPTER 12

Everyday ASMR

Now that you have a grasp of what ASMR is and how it works and have identified your triggers, as well as started using online content for rest and relaxation, you may be wondering if your newly learned ASMR techniques and practices have any application in real-world scenarios. The answer is yes!

However, you do not have to bust out the webcam or set up a YouTube channel in order to help others through ASMR techniques. We have identified several areas in everyday life in which ASMR practices can subtly soothe others, helping them relax and become aware of the tingles inside.

In this chapter, we illustrate the various opportunities in the workplace or your private life in which you can use known ASMR triggers to help someone. We also let you know when those triggers will help and when they can hinder, so you can learn when to apply them and when to avoid them at all costs.

In This Chapter

- How to infuse ASMR practices into daily life
- Picking up on context clues
- When ASMR sensations become a problem
- Everyday ASMR videos

ASMR: An Extraordinary, Everyday Occurrence

Even though ASMR experiences are intrinsically tied to everyday events, they are not everyday occurrences. Rather, they tend to be situations people have been in many times before that somehow become spontaneous events that hit the right nerve at the right time and make them wish it would never end.

KEEP IN MIND

The ASMR experience is an extremely subjective event, so there is no guarantee that using any or all of these tips will trigger everyone you come in contact with.

More than likely, you probably have caused an ASMR tingle or two in your life, even if you didn't know it at the time. Have you ever held a sleeping baby in your arms and felt her let out a gentle sigh of contentment? Even though she had been rocked and cuddled numerous times in her short life, there was something about the way you were caring for her in that particular moment that caused her to react as though nothing could get any better. Though we cannot prove it, chances are what she was feeling in that moment was something similar to ASMR.

What if you could conjure that same feeling every day in friends and strangers alike? What if the way you acted on a conscious level affected people on a subconscious level? What if it could lead them to an ASMR experience? Would you try it?

Well, you can; in fact, in some industries such as the health-care field, cosmetology, and massage therapy, this kind of personal care and attention is critical to vocational success. If you are ready to apply ASMRtist techniques to your everyday interactions, get ready to provide a little comfort and contentment while learning how a little TLC can go a long way!

Building a Better Bedside Manner

The late Maya Angelou once said, "I have learned that people will forget what you said, people will forget what you did, but people will never forget how you made them feel." It is the fundamental key to applied ASMR, and it all begins with the ability to build a better *bedside manner* and to empathize with others.

You've probably heard this term before in reference to the way doctors interact with their patients in a hospital or clinical setting. Bedside manner is a kind of body language that affects professionals' vocal tones, physical stance, openness, presence, and concealment. In the medical setting, it is this manner that can have an impact on how patients react to their doctor's assessment. Generally speaking, a good bedside manner is one in which physicians remain calm and reassuring toward the patients, offer appropriate forms of physical communication, and convey their patients' condition in simple but compassionate terms that can be understood easily.

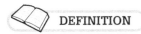

DEFINITION

> A **bedside manner** is the traditional way of referring to how a doctor interacts with her patient. It also refers to the caring way in which ASMRtists interact with their viewers.

However, the concept of the bedside manner goes beyond the health-care industry; in fact, it comes up in a variety of customer service–related fields. For example, cosmetologists and spa specialists (such as skin care consultants, massage therapists, and holistic healers) typically consult with their clients in order to help them feel comfortable before beginning a service. You can also see aspects of the bedside manner in hotels, restaurants, retail, and any number of other service-based fields where personal attention is at the core of the experience.

There are five main components that are critical to establishing a good bedside manner, and each plays a role in applied ASMR practices and techniques. Though some people believe that a good bedside manner cannot be taught, you can work on various components in order to offer your customer, client, or co-worker better overall service when interacting with you, no matter what kind of work you do:

- **Showing empathy:** You must be able to identify with what the other person is going through. Empathy is another trust-builder and one that can make or break the experience.

- **Maintaining eye contact:** This skill can help you establish a better bond with the individual. Be sure to keep your gaze gentle and your facial expression warm.

- **Listening:** Do not interrupt until the person has obviously paused. It may take the person a while to articulate her concerns. Be sure to hear what is said and unsaid (see the next section for more on reading the unsaid messages).

- **Sparing a moment:** Although you may have a schedule to keep, no one likes to feel rushed. Take the time to have a moment or two for someone who needs extra attention.

- **Touching:** If someone is already feeling very comfortable and relaxed, this may be the moment when you can trigger the tingles. Keep physical contact appropriate and sincere.

Above everything else, be true to yourself. This is one case in which you can't "fake it until you make it." People tend to see through insincerity fairly quickly, and if they suspect that you are being less than honest, it will not help you to create an atmosphere of trust.

TINGLE TIP

Although not everyone may respond to your mindful mannerisms, do not become frustrated. Stay calm in every situation. Not only will it help the person you are currently assisting, but also everyone else will feel your mood in the room. Keep in mind that you only have one chance to make a good first impression.

Cold Reading

Have you ever been around people who have seemed to know what you wanted before you ever asked for it? Contrary to what you may have thought, they do not have ESP or any other super power, and it's not that they have been around you so much that they simply "know." Rather, they are reading your body language for clues, comparing you to those who have exhibited those same attributes in the past, and making a logical assumption as to what would make your experience more enjoyable. In short, they are cold reading you.

Cold reading is a stage technique in which mediums, mentalists, and illusionists use body language, age, gender, and other clues to obtain large amounts of information about someone in a short period of time. It is a fairly simple process that looks impressive and yet is comprised of superficial facts and highly probable guesswork.

Some ways in which you can learn to cold read an individual include the following:

- Get to know the individual and find out more about her interests and hobbies.
- Ask open-ended questions and pick up on verbal and nonverbal cues in the answers (also known as "listening between the lines").
- Make appropriate assumptions about the individual based on the information that you have.
- Pick up on context clues that may give you additional insight into the individual.
- Delve deep to make sure you have all of the relevant information, and clarify any necessary details.
- Assess any needs and offer effective solutions.

For example, one of the masters of the cold read was the physician Joseph Bell, upon whom Sir Arthur Conan Doyle based Sherlock Holmes. By watching the way someone walked into a room, he could deduce a lot about the individual. A quick removal of a hat, erect posture, and the repeated use of the word "sir" could indicate the person had some military experience; a large knot on the ring finger near the nail may have indicated that the person was a writer; and a bruise on the chin just under the jaw line may have implied the person plays violin. There are a number of clues you can pick up on about a person when you pay attention to the individual's body language and mannerisms.

In many cases, the success of applied ASMR techniques comes down to whether or not the person feels that she has been heard and/or understood. Therefore, your ability to be attentive via cold reading will go a long way toward building trust with someone. Merely taking the time to listen, nod, and offer a sympathetic "um-hmmm" to show you care may be enough to trigger the ASMR sensation in someone else.

DID YOU KNOW?

ASMRtists cold read their audience all the time, though they do it through viewers' comments and requests. When they are researching material for their next segment, they think about what their fans want to see and look for opportunities to meet those needs in new and unexpected ways.

Proper Presentation

It's not always possible to predict what ASMR techniques will be most effective in any given situation. As you learned in Chapter 9, not everyone gathers information in the same way, so triggers are equally subjective as well. However, there are those times when actions speak louder than words. What tingle heads haven't had that moment in which they were triggered not by what a person does, but the way they feel when they watch that person do it? It may be the most ordinary task in the world, but when performed by someone else, it triggers the tingles every time.

In everyday language, this is known as the art of the *presentation*. Presentation is about enhancing aesthetic appeal. It is the difference between a plate full of food and a course that has been plated by the chef. The recipe may be the same, but somehow, it just looks different. Although it is commonly associated with the culinary field, presentation is applicable in a number of vocational settings, including ASMR. Generally speaking, it consists of two elements: the deliberate gestures that go into the process and the decorative end result.

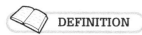

DEFINITION

Presentation is the art of modifying, processing, arranging, or decorating something in such a way as to enhance its visual appeal.

Although it occurs on an almost subliminal level, deliberate gestures send a clear and distinct message to individuals that they are in good hands. They are usually small portions of an overall action, but they are the element that goes above and beyond what people normally expect.

You can see examples of these gestures frequently in your everyday life, such as chocolates laid across a freshly turned-down bed, a receipt that is carefully folded into a little envelope, or an invitation that is so beautiful it could be a present itself. Even if you do not see the process that goes into creating the special end result, you are affected by the sentiment behind it. In turn, when people are able to see the loving, purposeful movements you made that signal an underlying commitment of care, it can lead to a powerful ASMR event that few people can describe coherently.

One of the best examples of how deliberate gestures lead to the ASMR sensation, as well as a decorative end result, is the "Relaxing Towel Folding Tutorial/ASMR" video by Maria "GentleWhispering" (youtube.com/watch?v=CHiKxytbCWk). In this 18-minute segment, she draws upon her skills as an ASMRtist, as well as a former hotel housekeeping specialist, to smooth, fold, crease, and handle linens in ways that few people do around the house. The result is a jolt of ASMR goodness for viewers, as with each movement she demonstrates how an ordinary event can really be extraordinary when performed with thoughtfulness and care.

You, too, can look for those opportunities around your workplace to add some ASMR actions to your routine. Do you work in a hospital or health-care setting and take the time to pull a sheet up or smooth down a blanket? That simple act of kindness can make someone's day. Did a client ask for a cup of tea? Bring out a small tea service and make it in front of them like a little ritual. Do you work in a clothing store? Don't simply show customers to the dressing room and leave them to their own devices. Gently assist them with buttons and zippers and help adjust the garments so they can have a better sense of fit when they look into the mirror. Do you work in a restaurant? Take the time to place menus, napkins, and other accouterments on the table in such a way as to convey that your customers are the most important people on the planet.

 DID YOU KNOW?

When you delight customers and clients with something extra that they didn't expect, studies show that they will very often reciprocate the gesture. For example, one study showed that when serving staff brought candy with the customer's bill, tips were higher.

We understand that everyone gets busy and there will be times when you can't slow your pace down, but when you take the time to demonstrate through your words, actions, and mannerisms that you are willing to go the extra mile for those in your care, it can result in increased business, happier customers, and perhaps a tingly feeling of relaxation they didn't know they could feel before they met you.

When ASMR Gets in the Way

While some people have to work hard in order to identify their triggers, experience ASMR, find content creators that work for them, and apply ASMR techniques in their daily lives, others come by it naturally. For the latter, there are therefore times when the ASMR experience can actually get in the way.

It is not always easy (or fun) to be a real-life, unintentional trigger for those types of people. When your natural mannerisms and melodic speaking voice causes an ASMR reaction in others, it can make for awkward situations. The most common is the ability to put people to sleep. We have heard countless stories of people whose friends tend to nod off in their presence (usually when they are talking), causing them to wonder if the individual is exhausted or if they are really that boring.

If something similar has happened to you, allow us to reassure you that you are not a dull conversationalist. You can also take comfort in the fact that there is something about you that the other person finds comforting and soothing and causes them to succumb to an ASMR experience. However, we do understand that that you may not want your friends falling asleep on you, so if you would like to retrain your voice so it is a little less tingle friendly, here are some things you can try:

- Change your pitch ever so slightly so your cadence conveys enthusiasm to the listener rather than relaxation. You can actually do this by smiling, as many people are able to "hear" the smile in others' voices.

- Monitor your pacing so you neither talk too fast nor too slow. Switching this up throughout the conversation will help people be less likely to become hypnotized by you.

- Consider your volume when you speak. If you are quiet, your listener has to concentrate more, which can lead to an ASMR experience. Try to be a little louder.

Above all, avoid rhythmic speech patterns that can be perceived as monotonous by other ears, and hopefully your pals will avoid visiting dreamland when they come to see you!

Another potential consequence of being an unintended ASMR trigger for someone else is being the recipient of perceived amorous feelings that arise as a result of the surge of hormones flooding the nervous system during an ASMR episode. As you learned in Chapter 1, scientists who have looked into the ASMR phenomenon such as Dr. Craig Richard have suggested that the relaxed, tingly sensation and slight euphoria people feel is most likely caused by endorphins, which stimulate a release of dopamine and oxytocin in the body. Dopamine is the "feel-good" hormone that results in an intense blast of alertness, improved short-term memory, the desire to explore the world around us, and a lack of inhibition. It is complimented by the softer, longer-lasting, and cuddlier hormone oxytocin, which is also known as the "love hormone" and is responsible for people being able to bond to someone else. When these two chemicals are secreted during an unrecognized ASMR event, the individual may project those feelings onto the person she believes to be causing them in kind of a "love at first tingle" moment.

This may not be a bad thing. If you feel the same way about the other person, by all means tingle on! We have certainly seen our share of ASMR love connections. However, it is far more common for those feelings to be one-sided and therefore requires the triggering person to defuse the situation before things become too uncomfortable.

It is not always easy to know if an individual's romantic feelings are ASMR related or not. However, if you know you have been a trigger for others in the past, you may want to listen for some key statements such as the following:

- "I could listen to your voice all day."

- "I immediately relax when I am around you."

- "You have a way of calming me down."

- "I love to watch your hands move."

If you suspect that you are triggering someone and you do not share their feelings, there are a number of things you can do beyond changing your pitch to resolve the situation:

- Avoid being alone with this person and stay in a group so that various voices and tones will merge with yours and be less likely to cause an ASMR reaction.

- Be mindful of the mannerisms and gestures that may be triggering the individual, especially if she has hinted at them in the past. Keep your hands in your pockets and avoid playing with your hair, touching the other person, or doing anything that could cause an ASMR spark.

- If all else fails, be frank with this person and simply tell her you are not interested. You do not have to tell her why you think her feelings are misguided (she might not understand anyway), and in many cases, it's enough to put some distance between you.

 KEEP IN MIND

If you are on the other side of this coin and are the one being triggered by someone you know, you don't have to be embarrassed by it. You are not the first person that this has happened to. Sometimes it is best to get the whole thing out in the open as a way to acknowledge the individual's effect on you and move on. By simply saying "Your voice is very soothing" or "I'll bet your kids love to hear you read them a bedtime story," you can mention their effect on you in a nonthreatening, appropriate way. That person may even be flattered!

Examples of Everyday ASMR

The following videos are examples of everyday situations in which people have reported experiencing ASMR. These videos illustrate how you may be able to use some of the techniques ASMRtists use in your personal and/or professional life in order to relax others around you or, in some cases, even trigger the tingles!

- **GentleWhispering: Relaxing Towel Folding Tutorial/ASMR** (youtube.com/watch?v=CHiKxytbCWk)

- **WhispersUnicorn: ASMR 3D Christmas Wrapping** (youtube.com/watch?v=uRppVPfCx_k)

- **The French Whisperer: Relaxation/ASMR—Wine Tasting Show and Tell** (youtube.com/watch?v=evPXPSYy1Do)

- **ShiverMeTingles: ASMR 07 "How To Find Flower Fairies" by Cicely Mary Barker—Story Time** (youtube.com/watch?v=0K8u6y2PgpU)

The Least You Need to Know

- You can infuse ASMR techniques into the way you interact with others.
- One's "bedside manner" is very important.
- Gentle gestures mean a lot.
- The ability to experience ASMR can be a hindrance at times for some, and there are things you can do to avoid being an unintentional trigger to someone else.

CHAPTER 13

Content Creation 101

Once you have found your triggers and become enamored with the ASMR community online, don't be surprised if you suddenly have a burning desire to join their ranks. Nearly every ASMRtist says they got their start the same way: giving back to the community that helped them feel less lonely, got them through the tough times in their life, or just helped them get some rest.

It doesn't take a lot of technical equipment to get started making ASMR videos, and soon enough, you can begin uploading your very own ASMR content on YouTube and generating a fan base of your own.

In this chapter, we explore basic ASMR content creation, with insights from leading ASMRtists on the secrets of their success and guidance through that all-important ASMR milestone: your first video.

In This Chapter

- Making your first ASMR video
- Developing yourself as an ASMRtist
- The equipment you need
- Deciding whether to be on or off camera
- Easy videos to start with

Getting Started

Are you planning to film your first ASMR video? Congratulations, and welcome! You are joining the ranks of countless content creators who have brushed, tapped, whispered, and role-played into YouTube immortality. Are you feeling a little nervous? Well, don't, because there is nothing to be nervous about. The ASMR community is a very warm and welcoming group of men and women who will be thrilled to have you on board, and it won't be long before you are connecting with many of your favorites who will suddenly feel like old friends.

Don't Quit Your Day Job

In order to get started in ASMR content creation, you need to ask yourself why you want to do this. If you have seen links to Patreon pages and PayPal accounts and have convinced yourself that this is a great way to earn some extra cash, stop right now. ASMRtists do not come to content creation hoping to make a fortune, and the idea shouldn't be foremost in your mind.

KEEP IN MIND

The income most ASMRtists receive through viewer donations is not usually enough for them to quit their day job, so money should not be your motivating factor for becoming an ASMRtist.

The ASMR community was born out of the idea of helping people and, for the most part, is a free service. Yes, some ASMRtists offer and charge for private Skype sessions, but the focus has always been and should always be on helping others relax. Typically, ASMRtists are compelled to make a video in thanksgiving to the content creators who have helped them get to sleep at night. And once they hit Record, they can't help wanting to make more.

What Kind of ASMRtist Will You Be?

Are you still interested in making ASMR videos? If so, the next thing you need to consider is what kind of ASMRtist you want to be. It is important to take a little time to stop and develop yourself as an artist so you know what kind of video you are best suited to film.

Although a lot of ASMRtists film a wide variety of segments based on current YouTube trends, fan requests, and personal triggers, most will say they have their preferences. While some current content creators like the sound videos that came from the first wave of content creators, others enjoy the *vlog*-style show-and-tells as well as the elaborate role-plays (see Chapter 14 for more about writing role-plays). There are pros and cons to each type of video, but ultimately it is a question about what skills you have to bring to the table and how your personal ASMR talents can be best showcased.

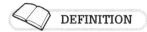

DEFINITION

A **vlog** is a video diary similar to its online written counterpart: the blog.

For example, if you have a shy personality and do not like a lot of conversation, role-plays and lots of whispering will probably not be any fun for you. However, if you are the kind of person who loves being onstage, dressing up, and pretending to be something you're not, feel free to open your own intergalactic travel agency, ambiguous medical practice, or virtual hair care center. Whatever the case, you'll get no judgment from us. This is your world and you can do whatever you want. As Bob Ross says, in your world, there are "no mistakes, only happy accidents."

Once you decide what type of content you're suited for, you should start simply. Although elaborate role-plays with all of the bells and whistles can be exciting and a lot of fun, current ASMRtists suggest that new content creators start small and become familiar with the process.

ASMRtist Robert "JustAWhisperingGuy" says when in doubt, new content creators should look around them and start with what they know and what they do. "My first role-play was a mixed martial arts hand wrapping role-play because I know how to do that from training," he said in his ASMR Day instructional video. "I do a lot of videos that have to do with things that I already know and for me, I think that goes a long way in seeming authentic and kind of flowing much better than if I were to try and research something and figure it out for myself."

As you can see from Robert's story, it's key to keep your early content simple and, above all, authentic. Do you have an interesting collection, a fun hobby, or a passion to share? Perhaps you work at a job that has interesting equipment you can show off. Plan your first video with this in mind; you'll grow into bigger productions in your chosen content as you become comfortable in front of (and behind) the camera.

Finding Your Voice

If you are planning to speak at all in the videos you make, you also want to consider the kind of voice you will use in the segments. While some ASMRtists still whisper, many of today's videos have segued to soft speech, which is a variation on the regular speaking voice.

TINGLE TIP

The worst thing to happen in an ASMR video is for the ASMRtist to speak in a voice filled with tension and anxiety. It is imperative that you are nice and relaxed so you will be able to speak slowly and with intention in order to get your point across.

As you know, the purpose of an ASMR video is to create a deep feeling of relaxation for the viewer, so when playing with your vocal range, choose something that is light and pleasant and that you can maintain without any sign of facial tension. Some ASMRtists say a good place to start is to test out the voice you would use to soothe a baby and go from there. You also want to make a point of practicing this way of speaking so it sounds as natural as possible.

Checking Your Surroundings

If you are thinking about filming your first ASMR video, chances are you do not have access to a fully equipped studio, scenery, or props department. It's okay. ASMRtists work from home all the time; however, they do have to consider the space where they plan to record and what kind of environmental sounds will end up on the final take.

The number-one complaint that content creators tend to receive about their work is the amount of background noise that appears in the finished product. While you do not have to stress too much about this or strive to create an environment of total silence, it is important to take the time to consider the space you are in and note any potential liabilities.

For example, if you live in a metropolitan area, you may have more difficulty with noise than if you live in the countryside. You also may have an easier time creating a quiet environment if you live alone than if you live with other people. Pets can also be a problem, as well as nearby neighbors whose kids may come out to play the minute you hit the Record button.

TINGLE TIP

According to Hailey "WhisperingRose," who published her first ASMR video on January 26, 2013, new ASMRtists just starting out should not spend too much time trying to create an atmosphere of pin-drop-like silence. "Sometimes that isn't necessary and sometimes people enjoy a little bit of hiss or background noise," she said in her ASMR instructional video from June 23, 2014.

None of this is insurmountable, of course, but it is one reason why you hear of so many ASMRtists filming their content in the middle of the night and in a closet so they can create as perfect a recording environment as possible on a limited budget.

In the end, some noises will be simply unavoidable. A sudden clap of thunder, a barking dog, a doorbell chime, or a phone ring—they happen! Every ASMRtist has had the same problem, so don't let it get you down or ruin your whole video. You can work around any noise.

Gathering and Becoming Familiar with Your Gear

Although ASMRtists often tout the various specialized microphones, cameras, and fancy editing software they use in the descriptions of their videos, you do not have to spend a fortune to start creating content. In fact, you may be surprised to learn that most ASMRtists got their start using equipment you most likely have right at your fingertips and reached tens of thousands of subscribers before making an upgrade (see Chapter 15 for more on equipment beyond the basics)!

In order to film a basic ASMR video, you simply need a camera (whether it's your phone or a video camera) and a way to steady your camera during filming. The best (and inexpensive) way to steady your camera is to purchase a tripod. These camera stabilizers with telescopic legs are incredibly easy to come by at yard sales and are not too expensive if you purchase them in a store or online. In fact, you can usually find them for around $5.

DID YOU KNOW?

On top of your tripod, you will see the camera mount—a small attachment that connects the camera to the tripod itself. While traditional cameras typically have a corresponding connection built in to the bottom of its casing, camera phones do not, which means you have to purchase an adapter for your model. These vary in price but are typically not very expensive and will enable you to stabilize your camera for the duration of your shooting session.

Once you have everything you need, you'll want to become familiar with your camera and its role in creating the experience. The first thing you will want to understand is where your microphone is located and what kind of sound it provides in order to create the best audio effects on your segment. Most camera phones do have a compressor on them and do a pretty good job of capturing sound, but some are better than others. Also, most external mics do not have a compressor, which means you have to be careful about how close you get to it in order to avoid the dreaded sound "pops" (such as the overpronounced "p" sound).

You will also want to understand how everything looks from your viewer's perspective and what you will need to do in order to offer them the best visual experience. Remember that what is shown onscreen represents what the viewers can see with their eyes; so if, for example, you offer them something to smell, you would not hold it up to the camera lens. That's not where the viewer's nose is located.

All of this takes a little bit of practice, and there is nothing wrong with preparing, rehearsing, and conducting a few test recordings to get the hang of it. You can then make notes based on problems you have incurred so that when it is time to film your first broadcast segment, you will have a solid plan in place to help everything run smoothly.

Preparing Yourself

While some ASMRtists do not adhere to any particular preparation ritual prior to filming, others find that it helps to try and relax their own minds before making ASMR content for others. There are endless ways this can be done, and of course every ASMRtist must find the system that is right for them. However, here are a few tips and tricks to help set the mood for your shoot, adapted from those used by ASMRtist Hailey "WhisperingRose":

- Put on soft, relaxing music to calm your mind.

- Turn off all electronics and portable devices unless you are using them for the shoot.

- If certain devices must be on, block all notifications for the time being so you are not interrupted.

- Take the time to get ready; select an outfit and put on makeup, if applicable, for the shoot. Your appearance really can add to your confidence level.

- Make sure the space you are shooting in is clear of any visual or auditory distractions. In other words, clean up any space that may show up on camera.

- Go over any notes you have made and mentally build a script for your video. (Some ASMRtists actually use a written script, which we talk about more in Chapter 14.)

- Test your audio and do a short test recording to make sure your equipment is working properly.

 KEEP IN MIND

Whatever ritual you engage in, be sure it is something that puts you in the right frame of mind for ASMR. The audience will be able to tell if you are not relaxed.

Ways to Film Your Video

Although there are several categories of ASMR videos and limitless props, story ideas, and sounds to help them come to life, there are only two ways to film them: in front of or behind the camera.

There are pros and cons to each option, and most ASMRtists do a little bit of both. But before you get started, you may want to consider how you feel about going public with your work and how anonymous you want to be. There are tingle heads everywhere, and it is not uncommon for content creators to be recognized in the oddest of circumstances, so it is important to think about how comfortable you are with being seen. The following sections take you through each type, as well as a way to do both.

Behind-the-Scenes Videos

Preferring to be behind the scenes doesn't mean you have to give up your ASMR career before it gets off the ground! If you are a content creator who prefers to remain anonymous, you can concentrate your efforts on off-screen whispers, nonvocal sounds, hands-only show-and-tell presentations, and even role-plays if you are particularly skilled at "talking" with your hands.

For your first video, we recommend starting out small, with something like a 15-minute, behind-the-camera, sounds-only segment, which is often the quickest and easiest type to make. All you have to do is to set up your tripod on a table, position yourself behind the camera (in order to see what you are filming), and go to work creating the sounds that will help your video come to life.

In case you didn't know, a sounds-only segment does not have to be silent, even though it is typically thought of as a nonspoken option. On the contrary, you can still include vocalizations in your video whether you choose to make noises with your mouth, perform an audible/inaudible whisper, or pretend to blow in your viewer's ear, among other things, while also tapping, scratching, scrunching, typing, or manipulating objects in order to produce sound.

Although you can choose as many sounds as you like for your first video, we do suggest that you begin with five sounds and spend approximately three minutes on each (you can check out asmrbebexo's sound assortment video at youtube.com/watch?v=_zf9jYJuq70 for an example of this type). In order for your viewer to have the best chance of experiencing the ASMR sensation, you will want to spend a thoughtful amount of time with each sound, but not so much time that it will become ineffective. You will also want to build pauses into the video in order to procure anticipatory tingles. When working with items, you will also want to take the time to show the object from all angles before using it to produce sound.

KEEP IN MIND

An ASMR video should be a multisensory experience. Therefore, even if you are creating a sounds-only segment, you can engage the visual and tactile senses with how you show and handle objects as you tease the auditory nerve.

If you'd like to get a better idea of how to do a behind-the-scenes video, some of our favorite videos in which the ASMRtist does not appear or speak include the following:

- **ViniVidiVulpes: ASMR Crispy Soundscape: Whisper Remix** (youtube.com/watch?v=6UrUsduW4FA)

- **whispersweetie: Hand Relaxation Number Two** (youtube.com/watch?v=wkXI5bGlCjU)

- **TouchingTingles: Binaural ASMR RP Ear Cleaning (Sounds Only)** (youtube.com/watch?v=a75P65gUaac)

- **SOUNDsculptures: 122. Playing Dominoes (3D Binaural—Wear Headphones)** (youtube.com/watch?v=kmPQO2R7odw)

- **oldwonderfulsounds: ASMR sounds (No Talking): Crinkle, Stickers, Paper, Plastic, Markers, Pens** (youtube.com/watch?v=FMeRrpq7d0s)

Face-to-Face Videos

Appearing on camera in a face-to-face video is a great way for you to connect with your audience in a deep and meaningful way. Viewers have the opportunity to read your body language, learn your mannerisms, and develop a quasi-relationship with you as the person who's helping them.

There is something very psychological about this idea and a reason that some face-to-face ASMR videos, such as doctors' visits and salon/spa services, are such popular segments with the viewing audience. Hairdressers, massage therapists, and physicians attest that there are few people in one's life that are invited to touch them or to care for them outside of family and close friends. When you re-create one of these events and assure viewers they are in good hands, it enables them to open up to the experience and relax without fear that you will take too much off the top, hit a nerve during a deep tissue massage, or diagnose them with cancer inside their faux medical practice.

TINGLE TIP

The key to creating a great ASMR speaking video is to keep everything you do natural and real. The audience can spot insincerity and will know if you are faking the experience.

As an ASMRtist, you need to be aware that this connection is being formed and it is not something that can be taken lightly. Viewers come to the ASMR community for a variety of reasons and whatever reason that might be, you are the content creator they are counting on, so it's up to you to give them your best. If you don't, they simply won't watch your video. Be empathetic, be supportive, and above all, be purposeful in whatever you do.

If you are planning a whisper video, it is important that you have an idea of what you are going to say to fill up the allotted time. Make sure that whatever you choose to talk about is something that will encourage a deep feeling of relaxation in your listener. For example, a guided visualization or meditation can be a wonderful way to introduce your talents to the YouTube audience (a sample guided visualization can be found in Chapter 4).

If you'd like some good examples of face-to-face videos to model, some of our favorite ASMRtist-featured videos include the following:

- **WhispersUnicorn: Whispering My Favorite Things** (youtube.com/watch?v=h_n4xOERr-E&index=6)

- **GentleWhispering: Relaxing Hand and Forearm Massage—ASMR Soft Spoken** (youtube.com/watch?v=DcfQY-0WwFo)

- **TheWaterwhispers: ASMR Soft Spoken RP—Personal Angel Card Reading Session** (youtube.com/watch?v=hW--56O1spY)

- **ASMRGRAINS: ASMR Male Grooming Session—Beard Trim and Haircut** (youtube.com/watch?v=PS4VBMshLMc)

- **amalzd: ASMR Relaxing Hand Movements (Softly Spoken)** (youtube.com/watch?v=Q328zHBikGI)

Hybrid Videos

There is one kind of ASMR video shoot you can do that is kind of a hybrid shot of the other two. It is a video in which you may appear onscreen, but your presence isn't central to the segment. Think of a cooking demonstration you may have seen on the Food Network: The camera is angled in such a way that you can see the individual preparing the dish; however, the focus is on what he is doing, not him.

As with any other kind of ASMR video, you can choose to speak or can remain silent for the duration of the film, but it is a different video from a close-up show-and-tell in which your hands may appear or a face-to-face vlog video in which your facial expressions and words are critical to the performance.

This kind of ASMR video is perfect for those people who are triggered by more visual stimuli rather than sound. It also enables you as the ASMRtist to use your hands in different ways, such as to make the slow, gentle, sweeping movements as you play with someone's hair, carefully and deliberately fold towels, make the bed, and so on. These kinds of shoots can be very effective and enable the audience to enjoy a different perspective.

If you're interested in trying to make a hybrid video, some of our favorite videos that demonstrate this technique include the following:

- **GentleWhispering: Soft-Spoken Relaxing Hair Play** (youtube.com/watch?v=OoNWLyNbFaY)

- **TheWaterwhispers: Comforting Whisper About Angel Hugs Dolls** (youtube.com/watch?v=Nce3xiekfBY)

- **MassageASMR: ASMR Creating Shapes with Kinetic Sand—No Talking** (youtube.com/watch?v=rlKD30xZh8Y)

- **WhispersRedASMR: ASMR Manicure and Massage—Olivia Kissper and WhispersRedASMR** (youtube.com/watch?v=cbTqqXhMtFw)

 KEEP IN MIND

Always know when to end your video shoot, and do not get upset if it is not as long as you planned. Sometimes ASMRtists grow bored making sounds with the same items for several minutes. It's okay; it happens. Be mindful of your own attention span and stop when you become bored with the sound. Trust us, if you have grown tired of it, chances are the audience has as well.

Editing and Uploading Your Video to YouTube

Once you have finished shooting your video, it is time to watch it, edit it, and upload it to YouTube.

We'll talk more about formal editing processes, equipment upgrades, and other filming tips and tricks from the pros in Chapter 15, but for purposes of a first video, we want to help you keep it simple.

To begin, chances are you do not have a lot of fancy editing equipment to work with, and that's okay. There are still a few things you can do to improve the quality of your completed product. You can easily use your phone's camera application to trim your video and take out the footage of you hitting the Record button or running around the camera to get into position for the shoot. (You can do the same to the end as well.) If you have filmed in parts and now need to put the pieces together, you can easily use simple computer software, such as iMovie or Movie Maker to create your collage.

There are a number of tutorials to help you walk through the process of making and editing a video using a variety of applications and software. Some that will help you perform a few basics include the following:

- **lynda.com: How to Shoot Video with Your iPad—Lynda.com Tutorial** (youtube. com/watch?v=m8_i6KY4ZdI)

- **trainingnpromotv: How to Film on Your Smart Phone or Tablet—The Smart Phone Video Guide** (youtube.com/watch?v=-QV6m1Z9Skw)

- **Kewkie Monstrr: iMovie Tutorial—How to Work iMovie/Basic Instructions (for Starters)** (youtube.com/watch?v=r8UzDHgm8rs)

Once you've edited your video, it's time to upload it. The actual upload process is fairly simple. We'll assume you currently don't have a YouTube account. In order to upload a video to YouTube, follow these steps:

1. Visit YouTube.com and click on the large blue "Sign In" button on the right of the page.

2. Fill out the form with all of your necessary information. (Use your Gmail account in order to save some time later.)

3. Choose the username that you want to be public, making sure it is one that reflects the ASMR image you want to present to the world.

4. Click on the acceptance of terms button.

5. If you used a Gmail account, you will be asked to link it and YouTube together; if you didn't, at this point you will be asked to create a Gmail account.

6. Once your account has been established and you are logged in, you will find the upload link next to your username. Click on it.

7. You will be presented with two options: to upload an existing video or to record a video. Choose the former.

8. A new window will appear in which you can select your video from your hard drive. Once you have decided which video to load, click "Choose."

9. As the video uploads, you will be kept abreast of its progress. While it is uploading, you can fill out the rest of the relevant information (title, description, and so on).

10. Do not leave that page until the video has finished uploading.

11. Once the video has finished uploading, it will take some time to process before it can be viewed online—typically anywhere from a half hour to an hour.

KEEP IN MIND

If you choose to upload your video from your mobile device, you may need to use the YouTube Capture application, which is a free application that can be found through your app store.

That's all there is to it! Once your video is ready for viewing, you will be able to watch it and share the link with your friends on social media.

Although the upload process is pretty easy, if you need further help in learning how to upload a video to YouTube, Derral Eves is a YouTube expert with numerous tutorials to get you started, including the following:

- **How To Properly Upload Videos to YouTube** (youtube.com/watch?v=Hlxqk0iHp5w)

- **How to Upload Videos Straight from the iPhone, iPod, and iPad to YouTube** (youtube.com/watch?v=TJmvXujqHNE)

- **How to Delete a Video from YouTube** (youtube.com/watch?v=p3j53oRXYF4)

The Least You Need to Know

- When deciding what kind of video your talents are best suited for, remember to start with what you know.

- You can make videos where you're in front of camera, behind the camera, or a mix of both.

- Keep your first video to around 15 minutes long. Once you get more used to the process, you can make your videos longer and more involved.

- Uploading to YouTube is a user-friendly process.

Creating Your First Role-Play

Are you ready to create your first ASMR role-play? Unlike the basic trigger videos you learned about in the last chapter, a role-play is a very different beast. A role-play is essentially a one-act production that must be planned and executed carefully in order to trigger tingles.

In order to create your role-play, all you need is a desire to write your own storyline, conduct the appropriate research, and rehearse the scene so that when the camera rolls, mistakes are minimized.

In this chapter, we give you the scoop on what it takes to craft the granddaddy of ASMR content videos. No matter if it is simple or elaborate, long or short, fantasy-based or centered around a real-life event, we help you fine-tune your creative muse and unlock your inner ASMR Shakespeare.

In This Chapter

- Finding inspiration for your role-play
- Creating the script
- Getting ready for your close-up
- How ASMRtist Heather Feather got into writing role-plays

Getting Inspired

Role-plays are some of the most popular ASMR videos on YouTube and some of the most unique. Although they started out as experience-driven segments centered on situations already familiar to viewers, such as medical exams, suit fittings, and salon services, role-plays have grown by leaps and bounds to include fantasy-filled episodes complete with elaborate props, costumes, and a variety of special effects.

If you are a longtime tingle head, chances are you have seen a number of these popular videos and have been inspired by their creativity. However, before you break out the camera and set up the tripod in hopes of filming something worthy of Steven Spielberg, it's important to take a step back and start small as you become comfortable with the role-play process.

The first thing you must consider when approaching your first role-play is what kind of video you plan to make. Are you best suited to present something educational, such as a cooking demonstration or a skin care session? Or do you prefer something more like a medical examination, which requires some familiarity with specific words and phrases? Will your video be heavily reliant on sounds and actions that can put your viewer in the hot seat of the experience, such as highlights or a haircut? (Chapter 11 gives you a rundown of some different types of ASMR videos.)

Regardless of what you are most comfortable with and what kind of video you have in mind, chances are there are several ASMRtists who have done something similar in the past and whose work will inspire your own content. To give you a starting point, here are a few role-play recordings to show you how the top ASMRtists started out and how they have developed their craft!

Heather Feather

- **Soft-Spoken Makeup Role-Play ASMR** (youtube.com/watch?v=Sqlo-_SoyHU)

- **ASMR After the Battle: Sci-Fi Suit Repair Role-Play for Relaxation** (youtube.com/watch?v=BR1WH6CpvRk)

ASMR requests

- **Cranial Nerve Exam—ASMR—Softly Spoken** (youtube.com/watch?v=Ae-c73J39KM)

- **Psychic Training Center Role-Play—ASMR—Soft Spoken, Ear to Ear, Tapping, Hand Relaxation** (youtube.com/watch?v=pBuXJSvvWn8)

TheWaterwhispers

- **ASMR Soft Spoken RP—Hair Stylist (Haircut)** (youtube.com/watch?annotation_id= annotation_590062&feature=iv&src_vid=kV_ZhyXHK1s&v=Xofvp6CxUkM)

- **Dentist Role-Play Appointment (Check-Up)—ASMR Most Requested Role-Plays** (youtube.com/watch?v=WF6bImb4G3w)

VeniVidiVulpes

- **Virtual Spa: Relaxing Haircut ASMR RP** (youtube.com/watch?v=2g9e2ner9sE)

- **ASMR: Paleontologist Role-Play** (youtube.com/watch?v=-Q-kTJiMN2I)

MassageASMR

- **Haircut Role-Play—ASMR** (youtube.com/watch?v=5RA5B2EHsJQ)

- **ASMR Role-Play—Dr. Dimitri Virtual Routine Physical Check-Up** (youtube.com/ watch?v=FWY9pVEE-SE)

Don't be afraid to revisit some of these videos in order to get ideas and make initial lists of the props and sound effects you would like to include. No one will call you a creeper; in fact, that's how other ASMRtists got their start as well.

TINGLE TIP

Although it can be great fun to create a completely original role-play with plenty of bells and whistles, veteran ASMRtists say that first-timers should start by modifying a tried-and-true role-play that others have successfully filmed. As you get more experienced and grow in the art form, you can create more elaborate segments.

The ASMR community is genuinely supportive of one another's work and tends to be very welcoming of new members. Established ASMRtists love when new content creators reach out to them, and they always appreciate an opportunity to talk shop with others. It's not uncommon for a member of the "old guard" to offer an encouraging word to a novice. They know what it is like to start out in the community and they are more than willing to mentor newbies along. Besides, even the top ASMRtists are on the lookout for new videos to sleep by, and who knows? Perhaps your video will become a favorite of theirs one day!

That being said, while it is great to have role models within the community and to find inspiration in their work, the goal is not to reinvent their wheel or to directly copy someone else's masterpiece. Sure, there might be some overlap between your content and someone else's video, but remember that you are an individual who has their own talents to offer the ASMR community; why strive to be a second-rate imitation of someone else?

Developing the Storyline

Contrary to what it may look like on the screen, an ASMR role-play is not a running monologue without any interaction between the viewer and content creator. In actuality, it is a two-person, one-act play that requires not only great characters, but also great character development.

The type of role-play you plan to film typically determines the characters that will be featured in the segment. For example, here are the ASMRtist and viewer characters in some typical role-plays:

- **Medical exam:** Doctor and patient
- **Tutoring:** Instructor and student
- **Salon service:** Stylist and client
- **Tarot reading:** Fortune teller and answer seeker
- **Interior design:** Decorator and homeowner

The list goes on and on. Once you know who your characters are, you must decide why is one seeking out the services of the other. Even though the viewer's role has no real dialogue, you as the ASMRtist must create something to play off of during filming to make the recording process run smoothly with no hiccups in the timing. You may decide that the patient (viewer) has recently experienced a head trauma and is in need of a cranial nerve examination. Perhaps she is a new homeowner selecting draperies for their living space. Or is the viewer a member of the wedding party getting her hair styled for the big day? While a role-play is not overly plot heavy, there is nothing wrong with adding a bit of a storyline to keep the episode interesting.

Choosing the Right Setting

Once you know what storyline you want to go with, you need to consider the setting of your role-play and where you plan to film it. When seasoned ASMRtists film their role-plays, they try to choose a space that makes sense for the kind of scene they plan to record and the character they intend to portray. They know that believability is key to the success of a role-play, and it may be hard for your viewer to open up and trust the experience if they do not believe the setting.

Chances are you do not have access to a fully equipped medical office, classroom, storefront, salon, or so on, so you may have to improvise a consultation space wherever possible that goes along with the "character" you are creating. Some ASMRtists secure background images and use a green screen in order to establish an appropriate environment, but most new content creators tend to use available areas of their homes, including their bedroom, bathroom, laundry room, closet, or office space.

In addition to finding an appropriate space to film where the noise level can be kept to a minimum and lighting is adequate, it is important to consider the décor of the area in which you plan to film. While you do not have to go overboard on set design or invest in huge amounts of scenery, a few small touches can make a huge difference to the overall experience. For example, you can invoke a medical examination room with an eye chart, a few diagrams, a clear container of cotton balls, and the presence of instruments lined up neatly on a metal tray. An impromptu classroom can be created with a map, a blackboard, and a few school supplies. And what spa doesn't include a few glowing candles for ambience? You'll find there is a lot you can do that will offer your viewer the essence of the experience without having to stage the whole event.

TINGLE TIP

When staging and planning your first role-play, keep it simple. Do not go overboard. It is very easy to get overwhelmed creating something time-consuming and elaborate to film. However, it's best to leave more intricate segments for when you have more experience under your belt.

Conducting Your Research

Once you have decided on your role-play and determined its setting, the next step is to study the event you plan to re-enact. Some ASMRtists research their role-plays thoroughly, while others prefer to improvise, refer to other videos, or rely on personal recollection for their video content. We feel the amount of research you conduct on your role-play is largely dependent on what the content is.

If you plan to film a makeup tutorial or a cooking demonstration, for example, there is nothing wrong with using your own technique, but a medical exam, craft how-to, or foreign language study session may require a bit more preparation to lend credibility to the final script. ASMR viewers are very sharp and know when content creators have done their homework and when they are making it up as they go along. Why not take the time to learn more about the role you plan to assume, watch the pros, and break down all of the elements in order to faithfully re-create the event? It will only make your video that much better in the long run.

Knowing the Lingo

Throughout your video, you are assuming the role of a character who looks, walks, talks, and acts a certain way, meaning dialogue is critical to your role-play's success. When you know the proper terms for the props you intend to use or invoke the nomenclature of the field you are pretending to be an expert in, it only adds to the believability of the set-up.

Think about the last time you walked into a service-based business. Did someone from the staff greet you? What did she say? If it was a situation where an appointment is appropriate, did you tell her what time you were expected and wait for her to confirm this information on a desk calendar or on a computer? Were you asked to fill out any paperwork before proceeding, or did you merely answer some basic questions about the purpose of your visit while the individual took a few notes?

Knowing the nuances of this exchange can help put your viewers at ease and prepare them for the experience that lies ahead. While you only need to master a portion of the parlance to pull off a role-play, many of these scenarios have their own terminology, making it important that you pick up on at least a few of the key points.

For example, let's say you are planning to film a cranial nerve examination. If you were to look up this particular assessment, you would learn about the parts of the body it is designed to evaluate and what problems a physician is screening for when she conducts it. You will also learn the actual elements of the exam and become familiar with terms such as *fundoscopy, visual reflexes,* and *olfactory nerve.* This official language and knowledge can give your video some extra depth. And if you take the time to study these terms and know what they actually mean, you will not only sound like you know what you are talking about, but it can also make your viewers wonder if you are a real physician.

 KEEP IN MIND

It is a good idea to add a disclaimer in your video description box to any medical role-plays that you are not a licensed clinician and that nothing you say should be taken as legitimate medical advice.

Simulating the Sounds

The trickiest part of the ASMR role-play is replicating the sounds associated with the service provided. Keep in mind, you as an ASMRtist are playing to a camera that does not have hair in need of cutting, ears in need of cleaning, or a face that needs makeup applied to it, yet you must find a way to re-create the sensations not only as they are performed but how they are heard and felt by the viewer.

To deal with this and gather more information about what will and won't work in a role-play, you should spend a lot of time tapping, scratching, and crinkling items next to your ears. Sometimes you may use the item to re-create a noise associated with a real-life experience, while other times the sound may become the inspiration for its own storyline. On occasion, you can turn to sound samples from internet sources when the role-play warrants it (freesound.org, soundbible. com, and pdsounds.org are good sources for sound samples), but nothing is ever off limits when it comes to tickling the tympanic nerve.

For example, ASMRtist Heather Feather is constantly testing objects to understand the sounds they make and how she can use them. "The way I interact with objects is different since I became a content creator. I tap everything I touch. Everything is a potential trigger source, and I am always looking for new things to use," she says. "My Candy Queen role-play came about when I went into a party store and saw a wall of candy and thought 'I want to use those in a video. How do I do it?' I am always brainstorming new ideas; it's part of the fun."

Are you ready to explore some of the sounds that ASMRtists use to execute their role-plays? The following are just a few suggestions for three of the most popular role-plays:

- **Salon role-play sounds:** Typical sounds used by ASMRtists in these videos are a water source or spray bottle, scissors, brushes, and prop product bottles. They also have a way to evoke the sound of actually brushing someone's hair. (This can be done by brushing a terry cloth towel or using a wig, hair extensions, or a doll styling head.)

- **Medical role-play sounds:** These sounds run the gamut, but many ASMRtists include latex gloves, a small penlight, and a small spray bottle (to mimic antiseptic cleaning). Some ASMRtists will even open real adhesive bandages to heal fake wounds because the sound of the thin paper is very distinctive and pleasurable to viewers' ears.

- **Makeover role-play sounds:** These videos include a lot of bottles, jars, and container sounds. However, these role-plays are most known for brushing sounds, which are achieved simply by ASMRtists stroking their microphone gently with makeup or artistic brushes.

TINGLE TIP

Looking for an easy way to re-create a scalp massage? Rub teabags between your fingers near the microphone to mimic the familiar scratching sound.

However, no matter what kind of sound sensations you plan to re-create in your role-plays, it is important that you know how your microphone picks up sound and various noises in the area that you plan to film. No two microphones are the same, so before finalizing your special effects, do a couple of test recordings so you are aware of how your equipment captures the sound. That way, you'll understand what you need to do in what way to record the sound you'd like to share with viewers.

Writing Your Role-Play Script

Now that you have your characters, know your basic storyline, and have done all of the research you need to execute your role-play, it is time to write the script. If you have never penned a script before, you are in for a unique experience.

Some ASMRtists prefer to improvise their segments rather than stick to any lines, but we feel if this is your first experience with a role-play or if you are planning something fairly elaborate, it may be wise to map it out in order to stay on track and keep the show running smoothly. (See Appendix D for an example of a full role-play script.)

Writing for Time

Scriptwriting is unlike any other style of writing because when you write a script, you are not only writing for content, but writing for time as well. Therefore, it really helps if you have a sense of how long you would like your role-play to be. While ASMR videos run the gamut in terms of length, it can be helpful to have some parameters in place. If this is your first ASMR role-play, we recommend limiting it to 15 to 20 minutes. This not only gives you plenty of time to execute a complete storyline, but also is not so long that it feels daunting.

The key to writing for time is not only in knowing what words you want to say, but also what actions have to occur. If you have never written for time before, try this exercise: Imagine you are going to make a peanut butter and jelly sandwich. How do you do it? The directions are much different than the actual steps. Do you start with the bread, or does the sandwich begin when you go to the pantry to gather the ingredients and then lay them on the kitchen counter? Is the knife already present, or do you have to take it out of the drawer? How far away is the drawer?

The actual directions assume you have everything in place and can start assembling the sandwich right away, but in actuality, there is a lot of action that is not accounted for in the process and it is this action that you have to be mindful of as you map out your role-play.

Composing the Introduction

The introduction consists of the initial interaction between your two characters. For this, you begin by welcoming your viewer to the experience and inquiring about the reason for their visit. It is the segment that sets the tone for the entire video and is geared toward establishing a rapport with your viewers so they become accustomed to your voice and the setting and will feel comfortable in your "presence."

For example, will you check their appointment in a datebook or on the computer? Will you be typing their intake information or taking it down by hand? How long should the pauses be between one question and the next? Will you stay seated the entire time, or will you get up from the chair and walk around? Remember that everything you do contributes to the overall effect and cannot be taken for granted.

An example of an introduction may include the following:

ASMRTIST

Hello there and welcome to (NAME OF BUSINESS). Do you have an appointment?

[Pause long enough for the VIEWER to answer yes.]

Great, can I get your last name?

[Pause to type in a name or check an appointment book for the correct name.]

And your first name?

[Another pause to ether type in the first name or check the book again.]

Oh here you are. I see you are scheduled for the (NAME OF SERVICE).

Penning the Consultation

The consultation is the show-and-tell portion of the role-play. It is similar to the beginning of a hypnosis session and helps the viewer relax even more fully in preparation for the sensory experience that lies ahead. During this segment, you will offer your guests an overview of what they can expect to experience and display some of the props that will be central to the performance.

For example, if you are performing a salon service, you might gently stroke the bristles of the brushes or tap the side of a shampoo bottle. If it is a medical exam, you might gently explain the upcoming procedure and conduct a general health assessment (a more in-depth Q&A than the introduction). If you are filming a tarot card reading, you might shuffle the cards and give the viewer a brief history of the deck. The ideas are endless.

While it's perfectly okay to ad lib a lot of your dialogue, simply creating a decent outline of the consultation allows you to have a general idea of what you want to say and how you plan to say it when the time comes.

The following is a sample consultation for a salon service:

ASMRTIST

Because this is your first visit to the ASMR Hair Studio, you should know that you are in for a relaxing experience that will begin with a gentle scalp massage, a hair wash, and a trim using the most natural of products and style for your big night out on the town. Let me show you some of the tools I will use on you today.

[Hold up brushes, combs, products, and other elements while tapping, stroking, or otherwise handling them to make noises as you demonstrate their purpose.]

Putting Together the Sensory Segment

The sensory experience is the heart of the ASMR role-play. In this segment, you will center your efforts on triggering the tingles of the viewing audience. Although you might click a pen or tap on a computer during the introduction or make a few sounds throughout the consultation, the ASMR experience kicks into high gear during the sensory phase.

The sensory segment is the longest portion of the role-play video, contains the most triggers, and requires the most planning. It is a combination of voice, display, sound, and action.

If this part of the video sounds authentic enough, viewers will be able to connect to it and trick their brain into believing that it is really happening. Not only will this bring on a wave of tingly goodness and cause them to fall into a deeper state of relaxation, it may even put them to sleep. And this is a good thing!

For example, a sensory segment of an ear cleaning exam might include the removal of earwax and may resemble the following:

ASMRTIST

Now, because I have found a significant amount of earwax impacted in your ear, I am going to use these alligator tweezers to remove it.

[Hold up tweezers to show the VIEWER and tap the ends together to demonstrate.]

Yes, this can be a bit uncomfortable, but you will feel better afterward.

[Move around to the side of the camera, as if to approach the VIEWER'S right ear. Take a household sponge and use the tweezers on it to mimic the sound of pulling earwax from the VIEWER's ear.]

 KEEP IN MIND

Be mindful of the components you will be able to successfully execute during the time allotted and which ones will sound the best to your viewer.

Scripting the Conclusion

The last portion of the ASMR role-play is the conclusion. It is the shortest segment of the video and the one that has the fewest triggers associated with it. This is where you will tie all of the loose ends together, finish the appointment, and wish the individual goodnight. While it is possible that your viewers will not even see this segment (especially if they are asleep), do not let the writing suffer at this point. Give it the same treatment that you do the rest of the role-play for continuity's sake.

For example, a conclusion for an eye exam role-play may include the following:

ASMRTIST

I am going to write you a prescription for your new glasses, which you can take to the optometrist of your choice. After that, you are all set for another year. But be sure to call our office if you have any problems between now and your next checkup. Do you have any questions?

[Pause long enough for the VIEWER to say no.]

Okay then, it was nice to see you again. Feel free to take your time to gather your things and see yourself out. Take care.

Gathering Your Wardrobe and Props

Once you've written the script, you should start thinking about the clothing and props you need for your video.

Although you do not have to go out and buy a costume (unless you choose to), you will want to give some consideration to what you want to wear during your role-play. Remember that unlike traditional trigger videos that are a little more casual in nature, the role-play evokes a different kind of ASMR experience, so it is important to maintain some consistency not only in the set design and dialogue, but also in the image you convey.

We recommend that you dress comfortably during the recording of your video, but that you wear something that makes sense for your character. Typically speaking, doctors, therapists, and other clinicians do not wear pajamas to the office. By the same token, tattoo artists, boutique clerks, and hair stylists usually have their own sense of style and are not afraid to show it. While you do not have to go overboard with your look, put a little bit of thought into what you wear and dress for role-play success!

After you have picked the clothes that will help you walk the walk of your character, it is time to gather the props you need to round out the role-play experience.

Some role-plays require more tools than others. In real life, the cranial nerve examination requires approximately nine different items but can be replicated in an ASMR role-play with a minimal amount of props. And a salon service can require a fair number of tools in an ASMR role-play in order to trigger someone's visual senses.

Some ASMR props can be found around the house (such as a penlight, cotton balls, hairbrushes, and shampoo bottles), while others can be generated from a computer (such as an eye chart, diagrams, and so on). However, still others are more technical and harder to come by, and that's okay. Nobody expects you to have a blood pressure cuff or other piece of machinery at your fingertips. Depending on your role-play, you may be able to fake the sound you need with another item or adjust your script to work around it.

Rehearsing and Recording Your Role-Play

For some ASMRtists, rehearsing and recording a role-play can be a time-consuming process. For others, it's a snap. We are going to assume that you are like us and fall somewhere in the middle, so in this section, we give you information on how to do a run-through and all of the final adjustments you may need to make before pressing the Record button.

Rehearsal and Final Preparations

Once you have put together your role-play, you may be a little overwhelmed by the amount of dialogue and direction involved, not to mention the props you need to use to execute the actions. Don't be! You do not have to memorize any lines or recite them as they appear in print while you're doing things. They are only there as a guide and to help you fill your time with an assortment of words, sounds, and actions. How closely you follow your script is completely up to you.

While some ASRMtists prefer to keep things fresh and natural and edit out any mistakes after the fact, others rehearse a lot and record take after take.

If this is your first role-play and you have limited experience with performing on camera, we recommend practicing in front of a mirror in order to become comfortable with your character, to better understand how to best handle your props, and to test the execution of any special effects.

You also probably want to test your facial expressions and vocal inflections prior to recording as well. For example, if you are a physician examining someone's inner ear, chances are one of your eyes is closed, your mouth is probably opened, and when you talk, it may sound slow and measured. It's the same way you speak when you are feeling around one of those hard-to-reach places in search of a lost item. Or if you are pretending to examine someone's scalp, you'll focus on the individual's head, wrinkle your brow, look concentrated, stay focused on your motivation, and not look directly into the camera. All of these little nuances will help you create a better role-play experience for yourself as well as your viewer.

When you have zeroed in on the elements that you know you want to include, the words you want to say, and the things you want to do, you can edit your script as needed. It will most likely be much shorter than the one you started with because you are more comfortable and confident with the segment.

Once you've done that, feel free to do one last rehearsal to make any last-minute adjustments, and then get ready for your close-up, because it is time to record.

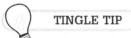

TINGLE TIP

Once you've rehearsed, you will then want to set up your stage, laying out all of your props in the order you plan to use them.

Recording

It is impossible to know for certain how long it will take to film your role-play. Some videos take a few minutes, some take a few hours, and some take a few days. It is largely dependent on the length and how elaborate it is. It also depends on whether you are interrupted by outside noise, if you stop for any mistakes, or whether you have technical difficulties of any kind. For example, some ASMRtists can film a 25-minute segment in 90 minutes with only a few hiccups along the way, while others prefer to refilm until it is perfect.

The important thing is to have fun with the process and grow with each video you make. Most top ASMRtists proudly display their first attempts at the role-play not only because it took a lot of work to accomplish, but it also shows how far they have come and how far you can go as a content creator!

My First Role-Play: Heather Feather

Known for her elaborate role-plays and cast of colorful characters, Heather Feather said she never actually planned to make ASMR videos, let alone become one of the top ASMRtists on YouTube. However, that all changed in 2012, when she suddenly had an overwhelming desire to record.

Like many other ASMRtists, she was motivated to give something back to the many content creators who had been helping her get to sleep at night with their videos. She rose from her couch, went into the bathroom, and filmed a 32-minute soft-spoken makeup role-play. She uploaded it to YouTube and the following day, she had six subscribers.

"I thought it was wild that anyone thought my video was worthwhile. So I kept going. I used my little point-and-shoot camera balanced on top of 7 cans of cat food. I didn't have any fancy equipment. I didn't even have a tripod. It was just my imagination, my memories, the camera, and me. It was the best decision I ever made," she said.

That first video took a couple hours to make. Now, however, her videos can take anywhere from 15 to 20 hours to prep and render. One of the longest she worked on was "After the Battle," a sci-fi suit-repair role-play that included Heather's first experiments with elaborate visual effects. She said that episode took several months to come to fruition and that the editing alone took weeks to complete.

As her videos have gotten more complex, it is Heather's hope that they have gotten more effective. Her goal is to have a huge variety of ways to trigger people on her channel in order to give people an escape when the world gets too loud. Heather says that ASMR videos have helped her immeasurably, and becoming a content creator was one of the best things she ever did for herself. "I would say give ASMR videos a shot … You can find a constant source of tingles, relaxation, and rest from thousands of individuals who each bring something unique to the table. Happy viewing!"

The Least You Need to Know

- ASMR role-plays are two-person, one-act plays.
- Some role-plays require more research than others because of the terminology (for example, medical exams).
- When writing a role-play, you are writing for time as well as content.
- Before filming, it helps to rehearse in order to feel more comfortable with what you're doing and get a more final script.

CHAPTER 15

ASMR Equipment Upgrades and Editing Software

After getting the hang of creating ASMR content and having a few productions under your belt, you may start saving your pennies for equipment upgrades that can improve the quality of your videos.

While it's no secret that some of the top ASMRtists on YouTube make significant investments in their gear to bring their audience the best ASMR content that they can, production equipment runs the gamut in terms of price point, meaning you don't have to break the bank to make an ASMR video. You can also think about purchasing equipment in stages in order to make it more affordable.

In this chapter, we walk you through the most common ASMR equipment and upgrades (such as microphones, cameras, and other accessories) and video editing software for ASMRtists so you can take the next step in content creation.

In This Chapter

- Binaural vs. stereo: which is the best microphone?
- Choosing the right video camera
- Extra accessories that add to the end result
- User-friendly editing programs
- Tips from the top: Ilse "TheWaterwhispers" talks editing

Sounds Good: Finding the Right Microphone

If you can only afford one high-quality piece of equipment for your ASMR production equipment, it should be a microphone. Although conventional wisdom would suggest that a new camera would be the best place to start, we know that sound is a critical component to the ASMR experience. Content creators can offer guided visualizations, role-plays, meditations, affirmations, and more without ever appearing on camera or adding visual imagery; however, they cannot do it without sound.

If you have ever taken the time to read through the comment feeds on ASMR videos, you know the primary complaint usually has something to do with sound quality. Though some ASMRtists are very popular without having the top-of-the-line microphone, sound is the one thing ASMRtists consistently strive to improve upon over the course of their careers.

However, with so many makes, models, styles, and brands on the market, where do you begin and what should you look for? Experts and ASMRtists say the first thing any new content creator needs to understand is *self-noise* and the signal-to-noise ratio. Self-noise is the background noise (for example, hissing and humming) that tends to come along with recording, making it an all-important factor when choosing a microphone for your video content. While every microphone in the world generates a certain amount of noise, some do a better job of reducing it than others. In order to find the best product to record your own content, look at the product's specifications; you want a microphone that has a low self-noise or S/N rate (15dBA or lower) and a high signal-to-noise ratio (above 80dB is preferable).

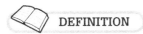

DEFINITION

Self-noise refers to the background noise that is picked up by a microphone, such as hums, hisses, and other distractions.

Binaural vs. Stereo Microphones

Now that you know what to look for in terms of noise reduction, you must decide if you want to purchase the famed binaural microphone, or if an omnidirectional (stereo) microphone will work best for you.

If you have been watching ASMR videos for a long time, you have no doubt seen a number of segments that include the admonition "binaural—wear headphones." Most ASMRtists swear by their binaural microphones; however, there is a lot of confusion as to what a binaural recording is and how it's different from traditional stereo recordings.

If you recall from Chapter 10, binaural refers to a sound recording with two microphones designed to offer a 3D effect. Binaural technology uses a multidisciplinary approach to sound recording that hits on aspects of physical acoustics, psychoacoustics, and auditory neurophysiology to produce a deep and lifelike resonance for the person who hears it. Unlike stereo recordings, which artificially split sound over two channels in order to offer the illusion of direction and perspective, binaural sounds are recorded using simulated headspace by outfitting each "ear" with its own microphone in order to capture sound the way in which people naturally perceive it. Binaural devices also include a membrane between the microphones so that when sound moves around the apparatus, the noise changes as it would if the audience was hearing it with their own ears in real time. (This is known as a *sound shadow.*)

While ASMRtists can produce a good-quality, ear-to-ear segment using a stereo microphone (or using two stereo microphones on either side of a dummy head), it is important to note that it is not quite the same thing. Binaural recording replicates key elements of the sound experience, and because it is recorded with the intention of being played back via earphones, it will not sound the same over traditional external stereo speakers. Therefore, we suggest purchasing and using a binaural microphone to create the best ASMR experience for your viewers.

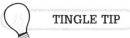

TINGLE TIP

Binaural sound is the reason why when an ASMRtist pretends to give people a haircut, it sounds the same way it would if they were in a salon. It is the immersive nature of the sound that gives it depth and helps re-create a real-life tingle trigger.

Power Connections for Your Microphone

Most of the high-end condenser microphones require an external phantom power connection in order for them to work. Phantom power is a term that refers to a method of distributing DC current through audio cables in order to provide power for various types of audio-visual equipment. This phantom power can come from a variety of sources, including recorders, mixers, and even your own computer.

Before purchasing your new microphone, you'll want to consider how you plan to record sounds. If you want to use your computer, you will want to look for a microphone that can connect via a USB port. For example, the Yeti (see the next section) is one such plug-and-play model.

However, most of the high-end microphones have XLR connections that are not compatible with a computer without an adapter. Therefore, a lot of ASMRtists forego the computer connection and embrace the freedom they get from a recording device that has an XLR input. The Zoom

H4N is an affordable solution to this issue, because it is not only a recorder but also has an audio interface and has its own high-quality microphone built into the system. It also allows you to use it as you upgrade your microphones in the future. It is truly a versatile device.

Best Bets for ASMR Microphones

With so many online retailers offering a wide range of stereo and binaural microphones at a variety of price points, it can be difficult to know which ones to look into. Luckily, you don't have to. Wendy and Paula, founders of the ASMR Academy, have experimented with and researched much of the best audio gear on the market in order to give new ASMRtists some guidance in their purchases. Their recommendations include the following:

- **3Dio Freespace Pro Binaural Microphone ($499; 3Diosound.com):** Used by a number of top ASMRtists, this microphone provides the best binaural sound.

- **Yeti Microphone ($120; bluemic.com):** This stereo microphone is considered to be the best value for the money and perfect for the newbie.

- **Zoom H4N ($269; zoom.co.jp):** This is a very popular microphone, recorder, and audio interface used by ASMRtists such as Ilse "TheWaterwhispers" Blansert, ThatASMRChick, and WhispersUnicorn.

- **Rode NT1-A Microphones ($550; rodemic.com):** This very quiet model is perfect for vocal recordings and podcasts.

- **SoundmanOKMII Classic Binaural Microphone (price varies; soundman.de):** This popular binaural recorder does well with panning effects (otherwise known as moving horizontally) that tingle heads adore.

- **Roland CS-10EM Binaural Microphone ($110; rolandus.com):** This microphone provides combined in-ear monitoring and binaural recording along with realistic sound.

- **Rode NT5 Microphones ($430; rodemic.com):** Used by MassageASMR, this model requires a matched pair in order to re-create his signature stereo sound.

Choosing a Video Camera

Although it is not as critical as a high-end microphone when it comes to creating ASMR content, a proper video camera can go a long way toward optimizing the quality of your productions. While some YouTubers get along fine with their pocket models and handheld varieties, others have made the leap into more professional video camera gear.

TINGLE TIP

Not sure when is the best time to start upgrading? YouTubers say that audiences are patient about upgrades provided the content is worth it and the creator is always striving to improve, but it's best to make some of the biggest changes after significant subscription milestones.

In general, there are three things to consider when purchasing a video camera: price, quality, and external sound capability. Obviously you want to buy a video camera you can afford without busting your budget. However, you also want to make sure the device is equipped with HD capability to give you the clearest picture available and allows you to attach your auxiliary microphone to capture the best sound.

Now that you've considered the basics, we'd like to take you through the different categories of video cameras, as well as some of the most popular options for filming ASMR videos.

Camera Categories

According to YouTube video expert James Wedmore in "Video Camera Reviews: How to Choose the Best Video Camera for YouTube" (youtube.com/watch?v=13MQKzDUUu8), there are three categories of cameras to consider:

- Portable video cameras included in smartphone technology

- Hand cameras or palm recorders

- DSLR

The first category refers to the portable devices that are included in smartphone technology, such as the iPhone. Wedmore says these are fantastic cameras for beginners because they are easy to operate, capture quality footage, and are perfect for use outdoors or in the studio (provided you have proper lighting). And considering you probably already have a smartphone, you won't have to shell out any money for one beyond your phone bill!

The second category is made up of video cameras like the GoPro Hero (gopro.com) models. GoPros are the size of a phone camera, are great for b-roll (rehearsal and blooper) footage, and are waterproof. Another hand camera Wedmore likes is the Sony Handycam (store.sony.com), which offers crystal-clear images, has an external audio jack, and has a manual dial to adjust the exposure of your video in the event there is low light in the room. Both types give you more control over the quality of your video and come with a lot of storage space (in the case of the Sony Handycam, 120 GB). Good-quality hand cameras like the two mentioned begin at about $300 and go up depending on the model.

As for the final category of cameras mentioned by Wedmore, DSLRs are typically the most expensive but have all of the bells and whistles and are used by professional filmmakers throughout the world. However, Wedmore says that there is a steep learning curve to using one of these models, making them challenging to work with if you are a one-person operation. As he explains on his channel, he recommends DSLRs "if you want the quality to be top notch but you have either a background in it, you're willing to learn, or if you can find someone who does have the experience and the know-how with these cameras."

No matter what category of camera you decide upon, remember it is not about learning something new (unless that is your goal); it is about creating video content as quickly, easily, and efficiently as possible. If you are not a technology buff and are nervous about learning something new, stick with your smartphone and improve your content with a tripod, external microphone, and better lighting (the latter of which we'll discuss shortly). If you have a bigger budget and want to make an upgrade but still feel uncomfortable with any special features, hand cameras are the way to go. But if you are up for the challenge and are willing to learn how to use it, consider the DSLR; it will give you the best visual result.

KEEP IN MIND

The camera does not make the content. We've all seen iPhone videos that have gone viral and high-definition segments that fall flat. Remember, the content is the most important component of the video, and not even the best camera in the world can save it if it lacks substance.

Some Popular Video Camera Options

In addition to Wedmore's recommendations, we scoured the web to find experts to weigh in on cameras that may be the best bet for ASMR content. The following are a few products that have scored big with reviewers:

- **Samsung HMX-W300 ($150; samsung.com):** This camera is cheap, has a built-in USB, is waterproof, and films in 1080p HD. This is perfect for shorter video segments.

- **Panasonic HC-V520 ($500; panasonic.com):** This is a "step-up" model that features a 28mm wide-angle lens, 80× zoom, built-in Wi-Fi, and a 3-inch LCD screen.

- **Canon EOS M ($649; canonusa.com):** Considered to be the best camera for the money, it has noise reduction and a touch-sensitive screen and can record in several resolutions.

- **Canon EOS 60D ($900; canonusa.com):** This is the preferred choice for many YouTubers who want a top-of-the-line product that can do anything without a top-of-the-line price.

Remember, even though prices may be a little better online, it's a good idea to go into your local camera shop and "test-drive" these along with any other models to see what works best for you. Sometimes these shops have trade-ins that will enable you to get a better camera for a lower price, as well as plenty of experts on hand with knowledge of several makes and models.

Lights and Backgrounds

While microphones and cameras are the "must-haves" when it comes to ASMR video production, there are also some "nice-to-haves" that can make your content pop. Who hasn't been impressed with an ASMRtist who has gone the extra mile with lighting and other special effects to create a segment viewers want to experience again and again? Although you can make an ASMR video without any of these added bells and whistles, if you are planning elaborate content or want to be on the cutting edge of YouTube filmmaking, you may want to consider investing in some of these items.

Finding Lighting Equipment

YouTube video makers say the biggest thing to take into consideration when filming a video is what kind of lighting is needed for the project. It's no secret that lighting is key to any visual image, but few photographers and filmmakers truly use light to the best of their abilities. We've all seen ASMR videos that have been shot by the light of the nightstand lamp, and while that does evoke a certain warmth, if you want to create professional-looking episodes for your channel, at some point you may choose to invest in some sort of lighting setup.

Think quality lighting has to come at an expensive price? Think again. For example, the StudioPRO 450W Photography Studio Continuous Lighting Two-Light Translucent Umbrella Kit (amazon.com/StudioPRO-Photography-Continuous-Lighting-Translucent/dp/B00FG5EVRW) offers two 45-watt CFL bulbs, along with two professional-quality aluminum adjustable light stands, two single-socket swivel AC fluorescent fixtures, and two 23-inch translucent soft light umbrellas for around $50 on Amazon.com. If you want to feel like a pro right away, a kit like this will do it, and those who have used the equipment have been pleasantly surprised by its quality.

Another affordable rig is the CowboyStudio Photography/Video Portrait Umbrella Continuous Triple Lighting Kit (amazon.com/CowboyStudio-Photography-Portrait-Continuous-Umbrellas/dp/B003WLY24O), which comes with three daylight CFL bulbs, three stands, two umbrellas, and one carrying case for the incredibly low price of $60. Professionals who took a chance on this easy-to-set-up kit have been impressed with the quality of the product and suggest that unless someone misuses it, it will serve a filmmaker or videographer well and have a long lifespan.

For those with a bigger budget, the Photo Basics 403 uLite 3-Light Kit (amazon.com/ Photo-Basics-403-uLite-3-Light/dp/B0028K2TWM) includes over 1,000 watts of power and is perfect for both the beginning filmmaker and the veteran videographer. This three-point set, which sells for around $250, comes with lightweight tripodlike mounts that are easy to set up and take down at the end of a shoot.

> **KEEP IN MIND**
>
> Lamps can get very hot during a shoot. Therefore, be sure to have plenty of ventilation available so your smoke detectors do not go off and ruin your take.

Backgrounds and Green Screen

Due to the up-close-and-personal nature of ASMR videos, some content creators do not worry too much about the look of their backgrounds, while others go all out and implement green-screen technology. Although it is entirely possible to produce a quality ASMR segment without it, we feel it is important to mention the different options available to you when it comes to background.

The easiest background to use, of course, is the wall of your room, provided it is a solid color or something that isn't too "busy" in terms of a pattern. Some YouTubers say a curtain or room divider can work really well and offers a quick and easy setup if you do not want to spend money to purchase one. If you do choose to make the investment, there are a number of background styles and sizes to choose from, including simple 4×12-feet paper backgrounds, printed versions, or fabric options.

But if you want more versatility and plan to do a lot of themed role-plays, you may want to consider making the jump into *chroma key photography*. Chroma key photography, or green-screen photography, enables you to replace a solid-color background (typically green or blue, which are as far away from our skin tone as possible) with any background of your choice. This technique has been used for a number of years in the film industry and has become quite popular around the YouTube community—and with ASMRtists.

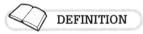

> **DEFINITION**
>
> **Chroma key photography** is the process of removing a solid color in order to replace it with any other image of the photographer's choice. It is usually done using a green or blue screen.

All you really need to film green-screen technology is a camera, your computer, your video editing software (see the next section for specific programs), and the all-important green-screen fabric. Prices and sizes of these vary by manufacturer and depending on your particular need.

Finalizing the Production: Choosing Editing Software

Once you have shot your video, it's time to edit your video and prepare it for upload. When it comes to editing and finalizing your video, one program does not fit every ASMRtist. While some content creators love to put on their editing hat and clean up everything frame by frame, others prefer the easiest and simplest method for getting ASMR triggers out to their fans. No matter whether you are a Mac or PC user, a complete newbie or a semiprofessional, there are programs at all price points and ability levels.

Unless you are filming an elaborate role-play that requires several takes and layers upon layers of sound and incorporates tons of special effects in order to achieve a seamless end result, you will find that editing an ASMR piece is fairly simple. It generally involves the bare minimum in terms of adjustments aside from cut-and-paste, adding titles, correcting color, aligning your external sound, and eliminating your extra vocal track. However, as ASMR production has advanced, some ASMRtists can't wait to pull out all of the stops with the latest programs that offer all of the bells and whistles.

In the following sections, we'll discuss the different types of editing software available to you based on complexity, as well as how author Ilse "TheWaterwhispers" edits her work. Don't be intimidated by fancy terminology; when you find the program that is right for you, you will produce your best work with it.

The Basics

If you are brand new to ASMR content creation, both Macs and PCs have simple, easy-to-use video editing software programs you will love. Apple customers rave about iMovie, an application that is installed on every new Apple computer and is perfect for someone who does not want to have a steep learning curve and wants plenty of templates to keep the process nice and easy. The PC counterpart to Apple's iMovie is Microsoft's Movie Maker, which is a free download for all PCs running Windows 7 or higher (windows.microsoft.com/en-us/windows-live/movie-maker). Users say the easy-to-follow instructions make video editing a snap, so it is a great place for the beginning ASMRtist to start.

Another basic editing program that has gotten a lot of buzz is Adobe's Premiere Elements (adobe.com/products/premiere-elements.html). This is a simplified version of its full-featured Premiere Pro but at a much better price point (around $80). It allows content creators to drag and drop video clips and offers plenty of point-and-click effects in the Quick Editing mode before taking it up a notch in Expert Mode. Other perks of the program include slow- and fast-motion speed effect, color adjustment, and options for sharing the final product on websites such as Vimeo. Experts say this program is a great choice for the ASMRtist who is beginning to make some upgrades to their equipment but still wants to keep things relatively simple.

Midlevel Options

If you're very comfortable with the basics and want to upgrade your editing software, you can start looking into some midlevel options. One of the most popular options at the midgrade level is Pinnacle Studio Plus (pinnaclesys.com/publicsite/us/products/studio/plus/), which offers ASMRtists an easy, user-friendly interface that is divided into three simple categories: capture, edit, and make movie. It doesn't get any easier than that! The program also enables you to control brightness, contrast, hue, saturation, and more throughout the entire editing process, which gives it an advantage over other options. With more than 1,500 transitions, effects, and other materials to work with (including green-screen background for Chroma key effects), you really can't go wrong. On top of that, Pinnacle Studio Plus also allows you to share your videos on Facebook, YouTube, and Vimeo. This software costs around $100.

Another midlevel program worth looking into is CyberLink Power Director 11 Ultimate (cyberlink.com/products/powerdirector-ultimate/features_en_US.html?&r=1), which is compatible with both Windows 64-bit and 32-bit OS. This program includes video capture, editing, and publishing options. It also comes with Content-Aware Editing, which automatically identifies important scenes and corrects bad footage; a 64-bit TrueVelocity engine, which allows for greater *rendering* speed; Design Studio tools; professional video effects; and complete 3D editing support. And at around $130, it is a full-featured option without the full-featured price.

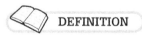

DEFINITION

Rendering refers to the process of calculating special effects into an editing program in order to produce the final product.

Finally, for many ASMRtists, Apple's Final Cut Pro X (apple.com/final-cut-pro/) is the ultimate in the medium-range video editing software. This program features visual simplicity and an exceptionally fluid, flexible way to cut and edit your work. Featuring a magnetic timeline, multicam capability, multichannel audio editing, clip connections, an inline precision editor, and an auditions feature to help you select the perfect shot, it's more than enough program to meet your needs. Reviewers give this program plenty of props and say that as the software has improved, it's only getting better and attracting a large number of editors from all over the spectrum. At $300, it's not cheap, but it's a solid program that will give you plenty of options.

The Big Leagues

If you want to be able to pull out all of the stops with your production, you can graduate to the big leagues with some high-level editing software. Sony Creative Software Vegas Pro 13 for Windows (sonycreativesoftware.com/download/updates/vegasprosuite) is a great place to start. Vegas Pro 13 offers creators a wide variety of features for the advanced amateur or professional filmmaker. Reviewers really like the program, though they do report that the upgrade from the previous model provided few new bells and whistles to get excited about. However, they do laud the company for balancing a powerful feature set with a beginner-friendly interface at a reasonable price ($399 to $799).

If you want to edit your work the way Ilse "TheWaterwhispers" Blansert and other top ASMRtists do, Adobe's Premiere Pro (adobe.com/products/premiere.html) is the way to go. Although it is slower at rendering than Final Cut, it is a program with a clean interface, flexible trimming tools, and plenty of organization helpers. It is a program that really gives you unlimited power in video editing and a program that you can grow into as you become more proficient with the process. This product is offered as a subscription service, with several plans available starting at $19.99.

Editing with Ilse "TheWaterwhispers"

ASMRtists know that even the simplest video can take a lot of work. Even if you forget the bells and whistles and concentrate on a natural segment without a lot of takes to keep the editing to a minimum, there is still a lot that must be done before your video is ready for YouTube.

The following are the basic steps Ilse "The Waterwhispers" uses to prepare videos on TheWaterwhispers channel:

1. Remove the SD cards and transfer the audio and video files to your computer and give each one a name.

2. Remove noise from the audio file and listen for improvements in sound quality. (This should take approximately 30 minutes depending on the length of the video.) You can check your program's features to find out how to do this for your particular editing software.

3. Import all the files into your editing program. (Ilse "TheWaterwhispers" uses Adobe Premiere Pro 5.5.)

4. Synchronize the audio with the video. This is easy if you snap your fingers or make another loud noise at the top of the shoot because it will be the only sound spike at the beginning; you can then sync the video with the audio from there.

5. Remove the audio track you do not need. For example, if you are using an external microphone for the "better" sound, you will remove the audio file from your built-in camera microphone.

6. Put all of the different clips together with simple effects, such as sound effects or a background image; when it is finished, listen to it a couple of times to make sure it is correct.

7. Add any website or channel information you would like to add in order to finish it off. For example, some ASMRtists use a title slide at the beginning of their videos along with a .gif or a signature tone.

According to Ilse "TheWaterwhispers," 25 minutes of simple content can take as long as two hours to edit, while complex role-plays can take much longer. She also spends another two hours saving the finished product before loading it to her channel on YouTube. (Upload times vary based on connection speed.) For her, editing an audio-only video is far less intense because there is no need to synchronize the video to it; however, if she uses a stationary image, the process is more or less the same, without the synchronization process.

"It's easy to underestimate how much work it can be to edit the audio and make it sound as clean as possible. A 25-minute sounds-only video can easily take an hour to edit, and if there were layers involved, the process would be much longer," she says. "Still, the effort is worth it knowing how much it means to my viewers."

So if you're moving into more skilled production work, Ilse "TheWaterwhispers" recommends purchasing editing software you feel comfortable using and meets your budgetary requirements. In the end, it's about not biting off more than you can chew. "The elaborate videos some ASMRtists are doing are amazing, but it's okay to keep it simple, too."

The Least You Need to Know

- Because sound is a critical component to the ASMR experience, you should invest in a high-quality microphone.
- Professional DSLR cameras come with a steep learning curve but provide the most professional look.
- Green screens and lighting are accessories that can really improve the quality of your work.
- Video editing software needs vary depending on how elaborate you plan to make your videos.

PART 5

Becoming Part of the ASMR Community

The ASMR community is a tight-knit group that is extremely private, so in this part, I give you tips on not only how to be a good audience member, but also how to best interact with others as an ASMRtist.

Professional ASMRtists are not only active on YouTube, but often have websites and blogs, seek promotion, and make money through ad sales and online donation/electronic payment sites. While it is unlikely that you will earn enough to retire on ASMR content, we show you how to take those next steps along the journey to a professional ASMR career. We help you strategize and market yourself in such a way that it will encourage new subscribers but not detract from ASMR's overall goals of rest and relaxation.

CHAPTER 16

ASMR Community Etiquette

It's easy to see why the ASMR community thrives on YouTube. The online juggernaut is the perfect platform in which to foster the symbiotic relationship between the content creator and the viewer.

While viewers depend on ASMRtists to create videos that will trigger their tingles, content creators rely on constructive viewer feedback in order to improve their work, which they dedicate countless hours of their time to produce. Everyone has a responsibility, and it is this kind of interdependency that can make a community stronger—or at times threaten to pull it apart.

In this chapter, we take you through some of the do's and don'ts of posting, watching, and responding to ASMR videos online so the experience can be fun and entertaining for you and everyone involved.

In This Chapter

- Staying respectful within the community
- Handling requests as a viewer and an ASMRtist
- How to best deal with negative people
- The importance of personal boundaries

How to Be a Good Citizen of the ASMR Community

When it comes to interacting with others in the ASMR community, "if you can't say something nice, don't say anything at all." It's a simple adage people were taught as children in the real world, but it applies to the YouTube platform used by the community as well.

YouTube is the third biggest site on the internet, and with more than 1 billion unique visitors watching over 6 billion hours of content each month, it may be the biggest thing to happen to the media since the internet was introduced to everyday people. The reason for this phenomenon is primarily the vlog—the online video diary that has created a completely new conversation that can't happen on the television platform and establishes a connection between the viewer and content creator.

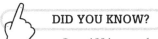 **DID YOU KNOW?**
Over 100 hours of content are uploaded to YouTube every minute.

It's no wonder that the ASMR community flourished in this space. After all, it is a phenomenon that is already extremely personal for those who experience it. Naturally, tingle heads have been thrilled to find forums and video platforms where the ASMR experience is shared, validated, and full of talented people willing to create free content to trigger the tingles.

However, even though the ASMR community is one that genuinely loves, supports, and cares about each other overall, it is a fact that there are some who derive pleasure from tearing others down and saying things behind a keyboard they probably wouldn't in real life. Despite what you may have heard about sticks and stones, words really can hurt—not only the content creator, but also other tingle heads as well. So to help you be the best citizen you can be, we've pulled together some tips and guidelines you can follow to get the best out of your interactions with ASMRtists and the community at large.

Being Supportive of ASMRtists in General

As you have discovered in previous chapters, it is a lot of work to be an ASMRtist. Many of these men and women have made significant investments of time, talent, and treasure to improve their content and bring you the best ASMR experience they have to give.

Contrary to what you might think, those who become ASMRtists are generally not seeking fame, and many have very introverted personalities. Through this art form, they have found their passion and they genuinely enjoy helping others find contentment, rest, and relaxation. They do what they love, and people love what they do.

Another misconception is that ASMRtists are out to capitalize on their channel. We will talk about the monetization of ASMR in the next chapter, but to be clear, no ASMRtist in the community has started their channel with the thought of using it to become rich.

Here are our tips for being a supportive ASMR community member:

- Do not pirate, copy, download, or use an ASMRtist's work for personal gain or promote it as your own.

- Do not call ASMRtists "attention seekers" or similar terminology.

- Do not put down the ASMR art form. If you prefer to be triggered through random experiences, that's fine. But let others enjoy their intentional ASMR videos.

- Tell your friends about an ASMRtist you enjoy. You'll drive traffic to that person's channel, which in turn will lead to more ASMR content!

- Subscribe to a favorite ASMRtist's channel and click on a few ads. ASMRtists appreciate the support, and it costs you nothing but a few seconds of your time.

- Do not compare one ASMRtist to another. Traditionally, ASMRtists do not compete, so stirring up a rivalry only makes you look bad.

In the end, it's all about being kind in your support of ASMRtists and the community at large.

Using Common Courtesy When Commenting on ASMR Videos

While ASMRtists welcome comments and feedback on their work, they really appreciate it when it is done in a respectful manner. For example, although not every video will trigger everyone and some are better than others, it's best to refrain from posting a curt "didn't work" or other unkind statement that could be offensive to someone else. Remember, no one person's triggers are more valid than another's, and everyone's feelings should be honored (including the content creator's). ASMR is highly subjective, and the nice thing about having so much diversity within the community is that there is something for everyone.

When commenting about an ASMR video, keep in mind that ASMRtists offer free content of a somewhat personal nature to help trigger their viewer's tingles, and unseemly comments regarding content or someone else's triggers is considered rude and should be avoided at all costs.

If you feel you must make a general comment about an ASMR video, here are the top 10 things to keep in mind:

- Acknowledge the amount of time an ASMRtist has spent making a video, even if it doesn't trigger you. Many spend hours on their content, so putting in a kind word about their hard work will help them feel it was worth it.

- The content creator may be experimenting with a new technique or piece of equipment. Even if it seems strange or doesn't trigger you, cut them some slack and let them get the hang of it; don't use the comments to complain.

- Rather than jump to conclusions about the video, ask about it. You never know what might have inspired it.

- You are not the ASMRtist's only audience member; you do not have a monopoly on the kind of content provided. Therefore, don't harass the ASMRtist with multiple requests or express dismay that the content wasn't geared toward your specific needs.

- Do not put down a trigger used in the video or claim "no one could be triggered by that." The ASMRtist may have been answering a request.

- Bracket any negatives with some positives. Nothing is all bad or all good. (But everyone prefers to hear the good.)

- Respect the fact that this is the ASMRtist's way of expressing herself and that you are being invited to share in it. Feel free to simply say thank you for their effort or for sharing their talent with you.

- Tell the ASMRtist specifically what you liked about a video. (Chances are, she will find a way to incorporate it again!)

- Keep your comments simple. ASMRtists hail from all over the world and speak many languages. Complicated comments may not translate very well.

- Don't compare one content creator's work to another. (Yes, we've mentioned it before but it bears repeating.)

Just by following these commenting guidelines, you'll show you can play nice with your neighbors and have respect for others, making you a good citizen of the ASMR community.

 KEEP IN MIND

No matter how hard you try, negative comments will happen. If you are a content creator, it can be hard to refrain from responding, but you must. Your best bet is to ignore their words and block them from your channel or social media site.

Making and Taking Requests

ASMRtists love taking requests from their viewers as much as their audience members love making them. It is a great feeling for the ASMRtist to know she has brought someone's idea to life, and tingle heads will tell you there is an added thrill that comes along with knowing they were the inspiration for a particular show-and-tell or role-play.

While ASMRtists admit they get some of their best ideas for content from viewers' requests, it is impossible to film everything that everyone wants to see, meaning decisions have to be made. Whether you're the viewer or the ASMRtist, it's important to know how to handle requests in the right way.

"I'm Still Waiting": Practicing Patience with Your Requests

We understand how disheartening it must be to feel as though your favorite content creator is ignoring your request. However, let us assure you there are a number of reasons why the content creator is unable to produce the video you have requested, such as the following:

- The ASMRtist does not have the resources or space to create the segment you would like to see.

- The ASMRtist has done something similar to it in the recent past and does not want to repeat it again too soon.

- The idea would take too much time to produce.

- It's not the kind of content the ASMRtist wants to put on her channel.

While we cannot speak for every ASMRtist on the internet, we do know that content creators strive to film the best episodes they can, with segments that are suited to their image. Therefore, it's best to respect their decision as final and not badger them with "reminders" that they haven't gotten around to your request or acknowledged your email. ASMRtists have noted that this kind of behavior is off-putting, sounds entitled, and does not make them want to honor the request in the future.

However, that doesn't mean you should never make requests. ASMRtists often have thousands of people to trigger and concentrate on content that will affect a wide range of people. In order to improve your chances of having a request made, consider asking for something that would include a lot of popular triggers, including taps, scratches, crinkles, and whispers. That way, you not only improve your chances of getting the content you like, you also give the ASMRtist a broader idea she'll be more inclined to use.

Being True to Yourself as an ASMRtist

But what if you're the one receiving the requests? If you are a content creator who feels over-whelmed by the number of requests your audience is making, do not feel compelled to try and do everything. Your fellow ASMRtists would tell you that above everything else, you must be true to yourself and make content that is right for you. Remember, your channel is your unique place of expression, so others should never overly influence it. If a request is not right for your channel or you are not suited for it, don't do it.

Still, one way you can honor a person's request without doing something untrue to you is to request it of a fellow ASMRtist. This is especially nice when you are a fairly established content creator and know of a new ASMRtist the idea might be right for. Not only can the request be honored, the other ASMRtist will probably be honored you referred it to her!

Dealing with Armchair Experts

While every ASMRtist would love to hear nothing but praise about their videos, they are realistic in the fact that some turn out a little better than others. If truth were told, most ASMRtists are harder on themselves than their fans are. However, every ASMRtist also has viewers who make it their job to nitpick over every distraction and point out mistakes as though an Academy Award nomination were riding on their assessment. It's not; it's YouTube.

Part of the fun of YouTube is creating that space that is all your own, where you can experiment with different ideas and put them out for people to enjoy. Everyone in the ASMR community is learning, growing, and developing their content to make it the best it can be; however, that does not mean mistakes won't occur from time to time or that distractions will not happen. It is very discouraging when someone feels compelled to tear a content creator apart or wants to argue with another viewer about the content of the video, and it only makes everyone miserable. We all have choices in the YouTube content that we watch. If you don't like it, you don't have to watch it, but don't play armchair expert.

That being said, constructive criticism is welcomed by ASMRtists, provided it is handled appropriately and as if you are not the source authority on ASMR content. (No one is.) Content creators love to know what worked for an individual and what they can do differently, but it's easier to digest suggested improvements when they come with a few compliments.

There are also moments when viewers come under fire from their peers for comments that they have made, even if those comments are made appropriately. Generally speaking, it is best to ignore negative replies to those comments and not to engage in an online argument.

Trolls

You've probably encountered *trolls* many times in the comments section of internet posts. These people love attention and thrive in public forums where they can stir up plenty of drama, and then sit back and enjoy the show. No matter how well thought of an ASMRtist is, all of them have or will at some point encounter a troll. So while it is very unpleasant to have to do so, dealing with them appropriately is necessary in order to keep your channel as harmonious as possible.

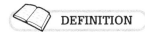 **DEFINITION**

In internet parlance, a **troll** is someone who uses the anonymity of cyberspace to start arguments and spread discord online. Trolls are similar to haters, who tend to be a little more malicious in their intentions.

First, if you are unsure as to whether your "helpful fan" with all of the advice is really a troll, ask yourself the following questions:

- Does she appear to be immune to rational thought and logical arguments and believe she is always right?

- Does she appear to like hurting other people's feelings?

- Does she refuse to conform to etiquette or simple common courtesy?

- Does she consider herself separate from the social order?

- Does she seem to gain energy when she makes you angry enough to respond to her?

If you answered "yes" to any of these questions, chances are you have a troll on your hands. The best way to deal with this person is to block her from your channel and all social media accounts. If she has access to your email address, flag hers and report it as spam so you do not have to deal with her at all.

On the other side of this, if you are a viewer who believes there is a troll commenting on a video thread, you have a few options. If the person's words are directed at your comments, you may block the individual or report her activity to the site administrator. If her words are directed more to the ASMRtist or another viewer and you believe this person to be a troll, you can choose to alert these people in a private message. However, once you do that, do not feel compelled to check on the status of that assessment, or offer to try and help. The worst thing that any viewer can do is to engage in a word war on a public forum.

Whether you are an ASMR content creator or viewer, do not let the trolls get the best of you! There are far more positive subscribers than trolls out there, and even if the positive subscribers do not post all of the time, they are always really grateful for an ASMRtist's efforts and the time they take to make ASMR content.

Haters

While trolls are on the relatively mild end of the hater spectrum, at the other end are internet grandstanders who thrive on using your platform or channel to post inflammatory statements and cause all manner of discord that goes far beyond the surface goading in which most trolls engage. Haters are cyber bullies who are determined not to like you and will go to the outer limits to annoy you. They will point out every flaw in every video and critique your looks, what you say, how you say it, and so on. They do not care if their words instigate a response or not.

There is a saying in the ASMR community that haters tend to show up when you are doing something right, and there is some truth to that. Haters typically do not bother with a new ASMRtist, but once someone builds her platform and draws in fans, they typically follow. While it's best to block these people and report them to IP administrators as quickly as possible, there have been a few cases where hating has gotten out of hand; in fact, a "cute bunny" became one of the best known casualties of the ASMR community.

CuteBunny992 was a 20-year-old Greek woman named Marianne who was living in Melbourne, Australia, at the time she began her YouTube channel. She was a natural ASMRtist who was known for her monologues in both Greek and English, as well as her youthful looks, which belied her chronological age. Longtime tingle heads can tell you she was one of the most popular members of the ASMR community until she disappeared from the internet sometime in 2012.

The reason for her swift and sudden departure has become a bit of an ASMR urban legend, but the known facts suggest that one of Marianne's fans became obsessed with her, stalked her online, and ultimately hacked the CuteBunny992 channel. In her video entitled "I am back!" the university student said that she believed the hacking occurred when she clicked on a suspicious link that appeared in one of her video feeds. The following day, Marianne received several emails alerting her that she had changed the password on her account when in actuality, she hadn't.

She immediately checked her YouTube channel, only to find out that someone had not only hacked it, but distorted the content as well. All of Marianne's ASMR videos were removed and in their place were videos that sullied her reputation and painted her in a bad light. There was at least one video that suggested she had an unhealthy attitude toward children, which was unfortunate considering she was studying to be a teacher, worked with children every day, and had mentioned in at least one of her videos that she longed to have a family one day.

Marianne sent out a plea on her Facebook page asking for help in reclaiming her channel and a few days later, she was finally able to return to the YouTube community. In her comeback episode, she said she felt like a phoenix coming out of the ashes and was looking forward to providing her audience with more content. However, it wasn't to be. After her explanatory missive, CuteBunny992 deleted her channel and deactivated her Facebook page, leaving some to wonder if the stalking continued.

A YouTube user named belaghouashi, who operates a CuteBunny992 fan page that broadcasts Marianne's videos, weighed in on the incident for the Matt Phil Carver Blog: "It was just one person being really annoying—aggressively so, stalking and actively trying to humiliate her. There were a small number of people … who encouraged and applauded him in this via comments on her channel when he still had control of it," he said. "Between the stalking and the … comments of those supporting it, she just decided it wasn't worth the trouble anymore."

However, on November 21, 2014, Marianne relaunched the CuteBunny992 channel on YouTube, to the delight of ASMR viewers everywhere. She said she missed the community but was inspired to return in part to Matt Phil Carver's blog, as well as encouragement she received from Emma "WhispersRed ASMR." Although she said she was still a little nervous to be in front of the camera once again, she was excited as well and promised to start filming more ASMR videos in the near future.

Marianne's ordeal is an extreme example of a hater taking control, but it's a powerful reminder of the importance of staying safe online, no matter if you are a content creator or a viewer.

> **TINGLE TIP**
>
> While the ASMR community lost one of its most promising on-screen personas, CuteBunny992's work can continue to be seen on fan sites. A couple videos you can check out are her cranial nerve examination role-play (youtube.com/watch?v=ZDZuaQ05Xso) and her hand relaxation video in Greek (youtube.com/watch?v=b77Mv_uPfUY).

Haters are a problem for other viewers as well, and although it can be difficult to ignore people's hurtful words and comments, it's best to do so for the sake of the ASMRtist. Sometimes, no matter how well intentioned, the viewer who gets involved is not doing anyone any favors by doing so. Trust us, it's like your mother always said, "If you ignore them, chances are they will go away."

Maintaining Appropriate Boundaries

While people like trolls and haters are looking to stir up trouble, there are others who seek an intimacy with ASMRtists or other community members to the point it's uncomfortable and even creepy.

While the definition of what is creepy and what is not varies somewhat depending on what the individual is doing, we define it as someone who has crossed the line of professionalism with an ASMRtist (or other YouTube artist/viewer) online or in the real world. Most fall into one of three categories: the superfans, the information seekers, and, for lack of a better term, the "pervs."

The following takes you through each type to give you more insight into how to deal with such people as an ASMRtist or viewer and what behavior is expected of you in turn.

Superfans

On the low end of the "creepy meter" is the superfan. This is someone who admires an ASMRtist and their work so much she cannot see them as anything other than a superstar.

Make no mistake: ASMRtists love meeting with and interacting with their fans, supporters, and subscribers. They know their channels would be nothing without them. However, ASMRtists are not celebrities in the traditional sense. They are ordinary men and women with jobs, families, and lives just like their viewers. The only difference is they have a camera and, on occasion, share their ASMR talents with the community.

We understand how exciting it is if Maria "GentleWhispering" or Ally "ASMRrequests" responds to your comment or returns your email. (Hey, we're fans, too!) However, keep in mind that their acknowledgment does not mean you are now best friends or that they will respond to everything you post. It also does not compel you to comment on everything your favorite ASMRtist says on her blog, social media, or YouTube channel. Being a fan is fine, but at some point you may be perceived as a stalker.

And if you happen to run into an ASMRtist in real life, please keep your excitement in check. Some ASMRtists prefer to keep their channel and their videos private and can become unsettled when they are publicly recognized. Many work extremely hard to protect their identities, so naturally they can become rattled if the person to whom they just handed their credit card or who delivered their mail turns out to be their "biggest fan." While ASMRtists are genuinely happy to meet anyone who appreciates the work they do, it is best to keep a real-life meeting as understated as possible (unless, of course, you are at an official ASMR event—if that's the case, feel free to get a little excited!).

 KEEP IN MIND

> If you do meet an ASMRtist in real life, do not be disappointed if she is not whispering or does not take 30 minutes to open up a box. Remember, many ASMRtists have developed an on-screen persona that is very different from who they are offline.

If you are the fan meeting the ASMRtist, here are some tips for interacting with that person:

- Be aware of the individual's body language to determine if they appear comfortable with being approached.

- Do not lean in and whisper "I know who you are." That is very scary for anyone.

- If the ASMRtist denies who she obviously is, let it go. Trust that she has her reasons, and do not send her an angry email/message about it later.

- If the ASMRtist appears comfortable with saying hello, be sure to say how much her work means to you and feel free to mention a favorite video. Everyone likes compliments.

- Do not expect the content creator to go into character or to ASMR you in public.

- If by chance you are privy to any personal information regarding the ASMRtist, reassure her you respect (and will maintain) her privacy.

- If you are in a situation where you may see the ASMRtist on a regular basis, only act like a "fan" once. After that, treat her as you would anyone else.

If you are an ASMRtist, chances are you did not begin making trigger videos in hopes of becoming a quasi-celebrity. However, if your work becomes extremely popular throughout the community, there may come a time when you are recognized in public, despite your best efforts to protect your privacy.

We understand that public recognition can be a frightening experience for an ASMRtist, especially if the individual is overly enthusiastic about meeting you, but it is important to remain calm and be nice and professional during the exchange. Also, keep in mind the following:

- Your fans help keep your channel going, so be congenial. Thank them for their support and be genuinely happy to meet them.

- Remember that your fans feel as though they know you. While you should always be yourself, be mindful of the "character" they associate you with and what they might expect when meeting you.

- Politely decline any photo opportunity or autograph that makes you uncomfortable.

Information Seekers

So far, we have not heard of any ASMRtist being stalked by the paparazzi, but information seekers may be a close equivalent. An information seeker is someone who has transcended "fan" status and is heading into stalker territory. These people are often longtime viewers who are a bit possessive about an ASMRtist and feel entitled to know more than everyone else.

They are the ones who try to figure out any little piece of outside information they can about you, trawl your personal Facebook page (if they find it), and send you repeated requests to connect. All of this is usually done under the guise of friendship.

Some information seekers are simply those who want to know more about you, while others are wannabe ASMRtists who want to get close enough to learn what you know so they can apply it in their own work. As you establish yourself in the ASMR community, it's simply important to guard your privacy and protect your boundaries.

KEEP IN MIND

The relationships ASMRtists have with their fans are real, and fans should trust that these content creators will share what they feel like sharing through their channel and public social media page. Beyond that, fans must respect their right to privacy.

From the fan perspective, we all have that burning curiosity about our favorite ASMRtists and want to know more about them on a personal level, but it is best to respect their privacy and allow them to tell the viewers what they want them to know. Prying for additional information will not endear you to the ASMRtist and will not cement your "friendship" with them. Don't misunderstand us: ASMRtists are generally approachable people who love to share their knowledge with someone new. However, they also believe in building genuine friendships within the community and are hurt when they feel used by someone pretending to be a fan-turned-friend.

"Pervs"

No matter how many times we reiterate that ASMR is not sexual in nature, and no matter how many times that has been confirmed by the scientific community, there are those viewers who cannot help making overtly sexual comments on ASMR channel feeds. This behavior is a solid 10 on the creepy meter and something ASMRtists wish desperately they did not have to endure.

There are obviously a lot of beautiful men and women who appear on ASMR channels, and there are those who may conceal their identities and only show the upper halves of their torso, their hands, and their mouths. This is not designed to be a turn-on, but to allow them to showcase their work their way.

While ASMRtists would prefer that people not make comments about their looks, if you feel that you must as a viewer, please keep it benign. Compliment how happy they look or how much you like their new haircut, clothes, nail polish, and so on—but do not turn it into something it's not.

If you are an ASMRtist who has been on the receiving end of such comments, the best thing to do is to ignore the individual. If their words get out of control, you can block them, but most ASMRtists simply feel that saying nothing is the best way to go.

KEEP IN MIND

Above all, try to understand if your favorite ASMRtist needs to take a break from their channel. Everyone needs some time off to recharge, including ASMRtists. Believe us, when they return, their content will be better than ever!

The Least You Need to Know

▪ Be a good citizen of the ASMR community by being kind to others and leaving polite, constructive comments on videos.

▪ If you're the viewer, do not hassle an ASMRtist about your request. If you're ASMRtist taking requests, don't try to be everything to everyone—stay true to yourself.

▪ Make sure to maintain appropriate boundaries with others. Don't assume a closer relationship with an ASMRtist than what's actually true; in turn, if you're on the receiving end, make your discomfort clear.

Going Pro as an ASMRtist

For some, the simple act of making ASMR videos as a hobby to help others and to gain a few friends along the way is enough of an incentive to stay active in the community. Meanwhile, others feel that ASMR is their passion in life and are ready to make it their full-time job.

We understand. When you hear about some ASMRtists gathering hundreds of thousands of subscribers, earning millions of views, and being recognized on the street, it's hard not to get caught up in the hype of what it is like to be a recognized "YouTuber."

If becoming an ASMR superstar is your goal, this chapter will help get you on your way. You'll learn how to establish the platform that will take you beyond YouTube and into the stratosphere of cyberspace. It's not an easy gig; there will be setbacks along the way. However, if this is your ASMR goal, this chapter provides all the guidance we can give to help get you there.

In This Chapter

- Setting up your own channel
- Setting yourself apart from other ASMRtists
- Gathering supporters and patrons
- Having the right attitude

TheOneLilium's Advice for Developing Your ASMR Channel

ASMRtists are both imitators and innovators. They begin by giving back their version of a favorite sound slice, whisper, show-and-tell, or role-play and before long, it becomes so much more. ASMRtists experiment with a mix of content—from the traditional to next-level ASMR experiences with production techniques that rival professional filmmakers—while looking for new opportunities to interact and support their favorite ASMRtists. In the end, many of these people create their own channels to share what they've made. What was a closeted hobby only a few years ago has grown into a serious career for some, and it's anyone's guess where it will go from here.

Are you ready to be part of it? If you are still producing ad-free content on your channel, using rudimentary equipment, and looking for your big break, we are ready to help with tips from a top ASMRtist.

Lilium, or TheOneLilium as she is known in the community, is a 20-something ASMRtist from Denmark who credits the YouTube ASMR community for saving her at a time when she was "not in a very good place" in her life and had a lot of trouble sleeping. After searching for some music or other soothing sounds, she finally turned to whisper videos, which eventually led to ASMR content. At a certain point, like others before her, she decided to make a video to say thank you to all of those who helped her. Nearly 100,000 subscribers later, she is one of the leading ASMRtists on YouTube.

In her video "How to Start Your Own ASMR Channel: 6 Easy Steps! Guidance and Advice" (youtube.com/watch?v=Dw9vbVbWVnA), TheOneLilium laid out her top tips for every new content creator who is considering their own channel (or who wants to take their channel further). We'd like to share and expand on some of the highlights from her video to help guide you on your journey to creating or developing your channel.

Get Inspired—and Get Started

Just as you looked to others for inspiration for that first video, you will want to look at other ASMR channels to determine what you want your channel to be and what you want to accomplish as an ASMRtist. For example, when TheOneLilium first started out, she was drawn to hypnosis and guided visualizations/meditations and saw that as her core niche. She therefore stresses in her video how important it is to find the place that will make you happy and allow you the chance to set yourself apart at the same time.

When you have an idea of what you would like to do as an ASMRtist, you need to create a channel name that reflects your ASMR career. While there is no right or wrong way to go about this, YouTube experts recommend using part of your name in order to make it easy for viewers to find you, and choosing a name that is distinct and does not sound like another channel.

> **TINGLE TIP**
>
> It is very easy for channels to get confused for one another. After all, there is ASMR Massage, amsrmassage, and ASMR Massage Psychetruth. Choosing something with ASMR in the title is fine, but it is important to distinguish yourself from other channels.

You should also take the time to make your channel a warm and inviting place for viewers to visit. Create a fun banner and choose a cool thumbnail that reflects the ASMR image you want to project to the world. Because online layouts are constantly changing (remember when Facebook pages didn't have cover photos?), it is important to keep up with your channel, perform routine maintenance, and check in with your dashboard in order to keep everything up to date; this will add to the comfort level of viewers visiting your channel.

Keep Lists for Your Channel

Whenever you have a new idea for a video, write it down. If you keep a running list of possibilities, you will always have a segment to shoot. It's okay if your idea seems unrealistic at the moment—write it down anyway! You never know where you will be in a few months or what you might be able to do. Challenge is good, so never be afraid to push the envelope with the content for your channel.

Another list you should make is one of equipment you may want to get in the future. As you have learned in previous chapters, it is perfectly fine to use the gear you have on hand, but there is nothing wrong with saving up for a better microphone or putting it on a birthday/holiday list. If your equipment is stopping you from moving forward as an ASMRtist, TheOneLilium says don't let it hold you back. She's been there, done that. "You can get a long way with a webcam and a headset microphone. You don't need to hold yourself back because you are afraid of not providing professional looking or sounding ... videos. That's not what ASMR is about," she said.

Get Comfortable with the Camera

If you are not sure what to do for that first video (or if you have only uploaded a few), make an introductory segment in which you introduce yourself and talk about what led you to the community. You can offer a shout-out to those who inspired your work, talk about your triggers, or discuss the kinds of videos you hope to film. Your "pilot episode" is all about getting comfortable in front of the camera and saying hello.

You do not have to appear on camera. Some of the most well-known ASMRtists did not show their face right away, and some never appear on camera at all—that's okay. Just have fun, relax, and always be yourself. The more comfortable you are on your channel, the more confident you will be in making new videos. This confidence will also grow when you start receiving glowing comments from your fans.

Interact with Others

The ASMR community has always been, and continues to be, a very tight-knit group. Although there are undisputed superstars of the field, it's a welcoming group of men and women who are genuinely thrilled to welcome new members.

For example, ASMRtist Olivia's Kissper ASMR said that when she first began her ASMR channel, she was curious to see if she could give others the tingles she felt and was surprised to learn that "ASMR powers" did not apply to a few people only. She said that although she understands the nerves that come along with creating a channel, just do it, and if you ever get down on yourself about your first efforts, remember to reexamine the first videos of your favorite ASMRtists and remember that they had to start somewhere as well.

"The community is so supportive of new people! This is one of the nicest things about ASMR. We are very supportive of people who are genuinely trying to create good content and less supportive of those who try and market themselves on other people's channels," she said.

 KEEP IN MIND

Under no circumstances should you post a link to your channel on another ASMRtist's feed unless you are invited to do so by that individual. We understand that everyone wants their channel to be noticed and to gain new subscribers. However, it is rude to bombard someone else's site with messages saying "Look at mine." It's always a better option to send a private link of your work to an ASMRtist you admire, thank her for her inspiration, and invite her to look at your work. Your fellow ASMRtist can take it from there.

When you have a channel, it is very important that you take the time to interact with and respond to your viewers. First of all, it's a nice thing to do when they take the time to write. Second, it creates a space where you can develop a one-on-one relationship with them. Third, your subscribers really can help your ASMR career in a number of ways. When you reach out to your viewers, they can give you feedback on your content, they can suggest ideas for new material, and they can keep you going when the trolls and haters threaten to get the best of you. Always be thankful and polite to your viewers and never forget that they are the people who are keeping your channel going!

You will also want to branch out on other social media sites—such as Facebook, Twitter, Instagram, and Snapchat—and build a web page that you can update from time to time. The more opportunities you create for your fans to connect with you, the better. Take it from us, their support means everything to an ASMRtist!

To Use Ads or Not to Use Ads

The idea of making money off of ASMR content is almost a taboo subject and not something that ASMRtists like to talk about. In the early days of ASMR YouTube content, virtually no ASMRtist allowed ads on their channel. This was not something anyone voted on within the community; it was just generally accepted that ASMR was designed to help people and should not be used for personal gain.

However, as the community grew, more and more ASMRtists began *monetizing* their ASMR channels at the beginning of their videos as a way to supplement their incomes. Opinions varied on this practice, but it seemed harmless enough. After all, becoming a YouTube partner does not mean an ASMRtist is making money based on the number of subscribers they have or how many views their channel gets. Rather, they make money off their viewers' interactions with the ads that appear on their videos. There are a couple of ways in which this income is generated:

- **Cost per click (CPC):** When an advertiser pays money based on the viewer clicking on the actual ad

- **Cost per view (CPV):** When an advertiser pays money based on the actual view—in other words, when an audience member watches the ad for at least 30 seconds or more

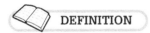

DEFINITION

Monetization is the way in which ASMRtists earn an income by allowing ads to appear on their channels.

Let's go over some options you have for advertising, as well as what you can expect to make by doing this.

Advertising Options

There are several types of ads that can be allowed on your YouTube channel, including the preroll ads that can be skipped over after five seconds and the in-search ads that show up as a viewer is looking for a specific video or certain type of video. There are also ad banners that appear at the bottom of a video (and only pay out when someone clicks on them), as well as in-display ads that show up in the suggested video listings while someone is watching another video. (There are also third-party preroll ads that cannot be skipped over by the viewer, but most ASMRtists do not utilize a lot of these.)

While you are allowed to choose the ad category you allow on you channel (such as health and beauty for a hair salon role-play video), you are not allowed to choose the actual ads yourself. You can also determine if the ad is shown at the beginning, middle, or end of your video, but because ASMR is connected to rest, relaxation, and sleep, it is most conducive to beginning or ending ad placement.

What Can You Make?

We've all heard stories about people who are making six-figure incomes from their YouTube channels, but we feel it is only fair to explain that you have to be among the upper echelon of content creators in order for that to occur. Most people who have monetized their channels (ASMR-related and otherwise) are not making enough to retire on.

According to a 2013 article by Carla Marshall entitled, "What It Takes to Make a Living from YouTube's Partner Earnings," most YouTube partners make between $.30 and $2.50 per thousand clicks (also known as CPM). Because YouTube takes a 45 percent cut of the money, this means the actual content creator is making only a fraction of that number on average.

When it comes to the top 1,000 channels Marshall found that they "bring in around $23,000 per month from advertising, but then again, they also average around 900,000 monthly video views, and because they're popular channels, they are likely commanding more generous CPM rates." So as you can see, it can be lucrative, but it requires you to have a large, sustainable audience.

> **DID YOU KNOW?**
>
> Some YouTubers are able to secure sponsorship and merchandising deals when they have large, relevant, and engaged audiences. These contracts are settled outside of YouTube and vary widely.

Getting a Paycheck from PayPal

While approximately 90 percent of ASMRtists have monetized their channels by allowing ads to appear, some have gone a step further and opened PayPal accounts (paypal.com) for those viewers who wish to make a financial contribution to their work. A PayPal account is an electronic merchant account that enables you to send and receive money while protecting the donor's privacy.

While it is free to set up a PayPal account, there is a 2.9 percent fee for each transaction plus 30¢ (in U.S. currency) for the amount received. There is no charge to transfer money into your personal account; however, if you prefer to receive a traditional check, there is a $1.50 fee.

The decision to solicit private donations is not without its controversy within the ASMR community. Some feel that ASMR content should be provided as a means to help people relax without any expectation of a reward; however, the option to benefit financially through private donations and paid subscriptions is something that many ASMRtists have taken advantage of. In many cases, the money earned from PayPal is used to supplement income or to upgrade equipment. If you decide to go this route, ASMR etiquette dictates that you place the links to any and all fundraising options discreetly in the description box underneath your videos and not overemphasize its presence.

Profiting from Patreon

The latest trend in which ASMRtists are generating income is through the crowdfunding site of Patreon (patreon.com). Although it is similar to Kickstarter and GoFundMe, Patreon is based on the patronage model of creating a long-term relationship between an artist and his supporters. Audience members pledge to support the content creator on a monthly basis and earn rewards based on their level of generosity.

TINGLE TIP

There is also an option on Patreon for supporters to contribute to their favorite artist based on the work they produce—in other words, to pay per video (usually $1). This is a great opportunity to make money on your work, but if you suddenly quit your day job and go full time, you'll want to alert your patrons that there may be a sudden uptick in production and give them the chance to change their level of support.

For example, a $1-per-month donation to an ASMRtist may give audience members special access to a supporter-only stream in which an artist may share some behind-the-scenes extras, interact with his supporters, or offer exclusive content. The next level (about $5) may offer supporters something a little more personalized, such as their name being incorporated into an ASMR video or mentioned at the end of a video. (They are also eligible for the lower reward levels as well.) ASMRtists are even creating private MP3 downloads, personalized greetings, and Google hangouts where supporters can spend time with their favorite channel host as gifts for viewers.

Patreon has not only allowed top ASMRtists to offer a unique service to their supporters, subscribers, and fans, but it has also enabled some to go full time, upgrade their equipment, and improve the art form. Naturally it is an exciting opportunity, and when you see some of the income ASMRtists are making, it's tempting to join their ranks. However, it is important to know when to make this move. Here are a few things you should consider before using Patreon:

- Patreon is an option for those who are ready to make a long-term commitment to their supporters and have the audience to back it up. Be honest with yourself about the level of support you already have. Is there room to grow where you are before moving on to something new?

- There is a huge difference between the top ASMR earners and the "average" Patreon ASMR incomes. Because many ASMRtists are using Patreon to campaign for donations, you could potentially get lost in the crowd, unlike the already well-established ASMRtists with larger audiences.

- Patreon is not to be used for equipment upgrades or one-time purchases. It's designed to be a subscription service, which means you have to be able to provide your supporters with the content you promise in return for their monthly contribution. If all you're looking for is a one-time monetary end goal, you can use Kickstarter, GoFundMe, or other sources more geared toward that.

- Do not sign up for Patreon because you think you have to. Some ASMRtists make a tidy income simply from their YouTube channel.

- Are you disciplined enough to juggle all of your ASMR responsibilities? Your main focus should be giving your time and attention to content creation, so think about whether joining Patreon will make things too hectic.

- Are you a brand-new ASMRtist? Creating a Patreon site right away may be misconstrued as being in it for the money.

- Will you be able to upload free YouTube content in addition to providing for your patrons? Never lose sight of what ASMR is supposed to be about: helping others.

DID YOU KNOW?

Some ASMRtists are using their Patreon sites to help eliminate ads from their YouTube channels. By making enough money from the individual subscribers, they can remove the ads from YouTube, which means that YouTube doesn't get a significant cut of the money. This allows ASMRtists to have more control over their income while giving their viewers commercial-free programming.

In the end, Patreon is a low-key option for ASMRtists to offer something "extra" to their fans; it is more of a destination site as opposed to a marketing tool. Plus, because it is relatively new, you may find yourself having to explain it to your audience. Keep in mind that ultimately, there is plenty of free ASMR content on YouTube, so if you hope to have your audience pay for something special, you'll want to ensure you are giving them the biggest bang for their buck.

Keeping Up With the Joneses

Because the ASMR community has garnered a lot of media attention lately and its YouTube content has been earning subscribers hand over fist, the time has been right for ASMRtists to take advantage of the opportunity that has been presented. Some have taken their work beyond YouTube and have worked hard to build platforms that reach audience members on a variety of social media sites.

That does not mean you have to do it as well. Just as you do not need anyone's permission to start your channel and create a segment, you do not have to "keep up with the Joneses" by monetizing your videos, starting a PayPal account, or launching a Patreon campaign.

The top 10 ASMRtists have built their professional platforms in very different ways. How much they earn from those platforms is a personal matter we will not speculate on; however, if you would like to get a sense of the network they maintain, the following is a breakdown of their activity and a link to their main YouTube page so you can see what they are up to. (Note: The top 10 varies depending on the number of subscriptions to the site, so we are basing it on the last published list, which can be found in Appendix E.)

- Maria "GentleWhispering" (youtube.com/user/GentleWhispering) is on Facebook, Google+, and Twitter, and accepts PayPal donations.

- Heather Feather (youtube.com/user/HeatherFeatherASMR) has a PayPal account; maintains a blog as well as a blooper channel; and is on Instagram, Google+, Twitter, Facebook, Patreon, and PixelWhipt.

- Ally "ASMRrequests" (youtube.com/user/ASMRrequests) is on Patreon, Facebook, Instagram, Twitter, and Google+. She will soon be launching a virtual reality channel on YouTube.

- Ilse "TheWaterwhispers" Blansert (youtube.com/user/TheWaterwhispers) maintains a website and is on Twitter, Facebook, Instagram, and Google+. She also accepts PayPal donations.

- Dimitri "MassageASMR" (youtube.com/user/MassageASMR) maintains a website and is on Facebook, Twitter, Google+, and SoundCloud. He accepts PayPal donations and is on Patreon.

- Ephemeral Rift (youtube.com/user/EphemeralRift) has a Patreon campaign and is on Facebook, Google+, iTunes, and Twitter.

- Violet "VeniVidiVulpes" (youtube.com/user/VeniVidiVulpes) is on Google+.

- TheOneLilium (youtube.com/user/TheOneLilium) maintains a website and accepts PayPal donations. She is also on Google+.

- asmrmassage (youtube.com/user/asmrmassage) is on Facebook and Google+.

- Pigsbum53 ASMR (youtube.com/user/pigsbum53) accepts PayPal donations and is on Instagram, Google+, Twitter, Tumblr, and Blogger.

Slow and Steady Wins the Race

Ultimately, the decision to become a professional ASMRtist is yours and yours alone. It will take a lot of time and energy, and success will not come overnight. But if you feel it is your vocation, you should do it; just be prepared to deal with both the highs and the lows of such a venture.

Amal Dabit, or amalzd as she is known in the ASMR community, said that having the right attitude is what keeps an ASMRtist going even if the going gets rough. For example, she finds it discouraging when content creators complain about the number of subscribers and viewers they don't have instead of being grateful for the audience they do have. "Even if you have 100 subscribers … who cares? Don't compare yourself to someone else because you will never be happy and you will never feel good. Wanting to succeed and wanting more viewers is good, but there are ways of going about it and, above all, being happy for people when they do well," she said in one of her videos.

So while it is normal for you to want more and it is good to always keep reaching, make sure you are thankful for what you already have as well. After all, you can't expect everything to fall into place all at once; slow and steady wins the race.

If you are ready to trigger some tingles and think you have what it takes to break into the top ASMRtists from around the world, what are you waiting for? We can't wait to meet you!

The Least You Need to Know

- Create the ASMR channel that is right for you. You want a channel that will make you happy and allow you the chance to set yourself apart at the same time.

- Monetizing by using ads on YouTube allows you to earn extra money in a way that's not dependent on your number of subscribers or how many views your channel gets.

- Play the Patreon card carefully. It is really a long-term option for the most established ASMRtists.

- Being successful as an ASMRtist requires having the right attitude. While you can continually strive for more, appreciate what you have rather than complaining about what you don't have.

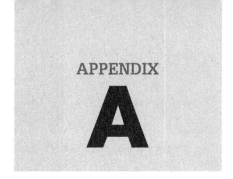
Glossary

anticipatory tingles   An ASMR term to describe the sensation people can achieve while waiting for the next trigger and not knowing when it will come or what it will be.

ascetic   Someone who practices severe self-discipline and abstention for religious or philosophical purposes.

ASMR immunity   A term used to describe people's sudden inability to experience the ASMR sensation when watching or listening to their favorite content.

ASMRtist   Someone who creates ASMR content in the hopes it will trigger tingles in another person.

autonomous sensory meridian response (ASMR)   A perceptual phenomenon characterized by a tingly feeling in the brain or scalp, which is caused by the experience or suggestion of external stimuli.

bedside manner   The traditional way of referring to how a doctor interacts with her patient. It also refers to the caring way in which ASMRtists interact with their viewers.

bilateral stimulation   A process in which someone uses visual, auditory, or tactile stimuli in a side-to-side pattern for therapeutic purposes.

binaural beats   A sound therapy practice in which two different impulses are played in opposite ears in order to produce a third "beat" in the brain that encourages a change in brain wave state.

biofeedback   A technique designed to enhance personal awareness and control over a person's physiological and psychological states.

braingasm   The term given to the tingle release that occurs during an ASMR experience, even though it is not sexual in nature.

chroma key photography   The process of removing a solid color in order to replace it with any other image of the photographer's choice. It is usually done using a green or blue screen.

empathy   The way in which individuals project their senses onto another experience in order to understand it on a cognitive level.

eye movement desensitization and reprocessing (EMDR)   A nontraditional branch of psychotherapy that uses traditional talk therapy and bilateral stimulation to help individuals cope with a traumatic experience.

hypnic myclonia   A sudden muscle contraction that occurs during the first stage of sleep and is typically preceded by a sensation of falling. It is similar to the jump that occurs when someone is startled.

hypnosis   The induction of a state of consciousness in which a person apparently loses the power of voluntary action and is highly responsive to suggestion or direction.

inner child   The aspect of a person's psyche and consciousness that is connected to and retains the feelings and carefree emotions of the past.

insomnia   A disorder characterized by a person's inability to go to sleep or stay asleep at night. It is usually diagnosed by a clinician because it compromises the work, education, health, and/or relationships of the individual.

lucid dream   Any dream in which an individual knows that she is dreaming.

mantra   A sacred syllable, word, or phrase that is chanted in meditative practices and believed to have spiritual, psychological, or healing power.

meditation   The act or process of spending time in quiet contemplation.

mirror neurons   Brain cells that cause people to respond equally to a particular action whether they are performing that action themselves or watching it be performed by someone else.

misophonia   The hatred of sound as a result of a condition known as selective sound sensitivity syndrome.

monetization   The way in which ASMRtists earn an income by allowing ads to appear on their channels.

neuroacoustics   A field of study that involves the direct application of precise sound applications in hopes of encouraging a physiological response.

neurotransmitters   The brain chemicals that communicate information throughout our brain and body and relay signals between nerve cells called *neurons*.

nightmare   A dream that occurs during the REM stage of sleep and evokes feelings of discomfort, fear, distress, and anxiety. It typically occurs in the latter part of the sleep state and tends to awaken the sleeper, who is able to recall various details of the dream.

nirvana   A peaceful state of mind that is free of ignorance, hatred, greed, and other desecrations.

posthypnotic suggestion   A suggestion made to a hypnotized person that specifies an action to be performed after returning to a normal state of consciousness, often in response to a trigger or cue. For example, if a hypnotist is helping someone get a more restful sleep, he might say "You will sleep peacefully with pleasant dreams."

presentation   The art of modifying, processing, arranging, or decorating something in such a way as to enhance its visual appeal.

psychophysiological   Refers to the combination of the mental and physical processes.

rendering   The process of calculating special effects into an editing program in order to produce the final product.

role-play   An artificial scenario designed to re-create a real or imagined situation.

self-noise   Refers to the background noise picked up by a microphone, such as hums, hisses, and other distractions.

stress   The physical and emotional reaction to the changes and challenges that affect individuals on a daily basis.

tactile-acoustic trigger   A touch-based sensation that results in a pleasurable sound (for example, popping bubble wrap, tapping fingers, clicking blocks together, shuffling cards, and so on).

telomerase   The enzyme that can repair the damage stress causes to the telomere, lengthen it, and slow the aging process.

telomeres   Genetic structures that serve as an end cap on the chromosomes and shorten as people age.

thermistor   A device used for measuring body temperature as it applies to an individual's stress level.

tingle head   A colloquial name for someone who experiences ASMR.

trigger   The stimulus that causes the ASMR feeling to occur.

tripod   A three-legged stabilizer that attaches to the camera so the photographer does not shake the image while he is filming.

troll   Someone who uses the anonymity of cyberspace to start arguments and spread discord online. Trolls are similar to haters, who tend to be a little more malicious in their intentions.

visual trigger   A stimulus that can lead to an ASMR episode when someone stares at it for a period of time.

vlog   A video diary similar to its online written counterpart, the blog.

whisper   A pronounced means of communication that is emitted through the mouth but does not require the vocal chords to vibrate.

white noise   A collection of sound vibrations that contain all known frequencies and result in a pitchless nothingness, which is used to mask other sounds.

Bibliography

amalzd. "Should I Do Videos/Starting Off In ASMR Community," YouTube video, 11:05. May 5, 2012, youtube.com/watch?v=3SoSTtfsenw.

American Sleep Association. "What is Sleep?" July 25, 2014, sleepassociation.org/patients-general-public/what-is-sleep/.

Anxiety Release. "What is Bilateral Stimulation?" October 18, 2014, anxietyreleaseapp.com/what-is-bilateral-stimulation/.

araniel. "Nova scienceNOW: 1—Mirror Neurons," YouTube video, 13:50. PBS, January 1, 2005, youtube.com/watch?v=Xmx1qPyo8Ks.

Artwork, Paul. "Research on the top 100 most viewed ASMRtists channels (not an ASMR video)," YouTube video, 32:14. June 20, 2014, youtube.com/watch?v=upUNzYKdJTI.

ASMR Research Organization. July 5, 2014, ASMR-research.org.

ASMRacademy.com. October 15, 2014.

ASMRlab.com. July 5, 2014.

Audira. "Hearing for Communication (and Interaction)." January 20, 2013, audira.org.uk/en/modernising-attitudes-to-hearing-care/item/19-hearing-for-communication-and-interaction.

"Autogenic Relaxation." October 1, 2014, stress-relief-tools.com/autogenic-relaxation.html.

Bair, Asatar. "8 Basic Kinds of Meditation (And Why You Should Meditate On Your Heart)." University of the Heart. June 12, 2010, iam-u.org/index.php/8-basic-kinds-of-meditation-and-why-you-should-meditate-on-your-heart.

Berkman, Randy, PhD. "Little Known Keys to Relaxation: Experiencing Healing Flows of Energy Throughout Your Body." *The New York Times,* February 1989, angelfire.com/pq/prophits/article.html.

The Better Sleep Council. "Insomnia." July 7, 2014, bettersleep.org/better-sleep/sleep-disorders/insomnia/.

"Biofeedback History." October 1, 2014, stress-relief-tools.com/biofeedback-history.html.

"Biofeedback Techniques." October 1, 2014, stress-relief-tools.com/biofeedback-techniques.html.

Blansert, Ilse. "Why do we experience ASMR?" TheWaterwhispers, July 25, 2014, thewaterwhispers.com/index.php/all-articles/92-why-do-we-experience-asmr.

Bringley, Krista. "EMDR Explained!" Life Skills Resource Group, October 1, 2013, lifeskillsresourcegroup.com/emdr-explained/.

Byrd, Ayana. "The Power of Touch." *Good Housekeeping,* October 15, 2014, goodhousekeeping.com/health/wellness/health-benefits-of-touch.

CalSouthern Psychology. "EMDR—Eye Movement Desensitization and Processing—20/20 Report," YouTube video, 11:30. January 27, 2012, youtube.com/watch?v=GTLLfdcJE0Q.

ChangeWorks Hypnosis Center. August 20, 2014, mn-hypnosis.com/HomePage.html.

Cherry, Kendra. "Why Do We Dream? Top Dream Theories." About.com, July 15, 2014, psychology.about.com/od/statesofconsciousness/p/dream-theories.htm.

Cohen, Joyce. "When a Chomp or a Slurp Is a Trigger for Outrage." *The New York Times,* September 5, 2011, nytimes.com/2011/09/06/health/06annoy.html.

Cohen, Michael. "How To Use Self-Hypnosis To Achieve Your Goals." Michael Cohen's Therapy Service, August 19, 2014, hypnosisandhealing.co.uk/self-help-centre/how-to-use-self-hypnosis-to-achieve-your-goals/.

Cramer, Kelly. "How Does Meditation Work." Project-meditation.org, August 5, 2014, project-meditation.org/wim/how_does_meditation_work.html.

Davis, Linsey. "Sleep Made Easier for Some Through YouTube videos." *ABC News,* February 25, 2014, abcnews.go.com/blogs/health/2014/02/25/sleep-made-easier-for-some-through-youtube-videos/.

Division of Sleep Medicine at Harvard Medical School. "Why Do We Sleep, Anyway?" December 18, 2007, healthysleep.med.harvard.edu/healthy/matters/benefits-of-sleep/why-do-we-sleep.

Dobson, Andrew. "About Binaural Beats." Mindfit Hypnosis, September 25, 2014, mindfithypnosis.com/about-binaural-beats.

Doolittle, Erin. "EMDR Part II." Anxiety Social Net, August 16, 2012, anxietysocialnet.com/therapists-blog/item/677-what-to-expect-for-your-emdr-session.

Dr. Oz. "The Internet's Crazy New Cure for Insomnia, Pt 1," online video, 4:08. April 10, 2014, doctoroz.com/episode/famous-deaths-reexamined-princess-diana?video_id=3453126244001.

Ehrlich, Stephen D., NMD. "Biofeedback." University of Maryland Medical Center, May 7, 2013, umm.edu/health/medical/altmed/treatment/biofeedback#ixzz3EtZRP17u.

"Feel More ASMR." October 5, 2014, feelmoreasmr.com.

Fernandez, Elizabeth. "Lifestyle Changes May Lengthen Telomeres, A Measure of Cell Aging." University of California San Francisco, September 16, 2013, ucsf.edu/news/2013/09/108886/lifestyle-changes-may-lengthen-telomeres-measure-cell-aging.

"Franz Anton Mesmer." September 1, 2014, anton-mesmer.com.

Freud, Sigmund. *The Interpretation of Dreams.* 1900. Reprint, New York: Psychology Today, 2013.

Hardy-Holley Team. "History of Hypnosis: A Brief History of Hypnosis." July 25, 2014, hardy-holley.com/history-of-hypnosis.

Harris, Tom. "How Hypnosis Works." HowStuffWorks, August 10, 2001, science.howstuffworks.com/science-vs-myth/extrasensory-perceptions/hypnosis2.htm.

Harvey, Richard. "Coping With Stress—Biofeedback: Self-Mastery Beyond Pills." UCSF Mini Medical School for the Public University of California Television, YouTube video, 1:28:41. March 2008, youtube.com/watch?v=iup0msVJeAI.

Hingston, Sandy. "Why Is Everyone in Philadelphia So Stressed?" *Philadelphia Magazine,* April 25, 2014, phillymag.com/articles/stress-in-philadelphia/.

Huffington Post. "Is This Why Some People Are Able to Remember Their Dreams Better Than Others?" Feb 21, 2014, huffingtonpost.com/2014/02/21/remember-dreams-brain_n_4809360.html.

Jarrett, Christian. "A Calm Look at the Most Hyped Concept in Neuroscience—Mirror Neurons." *Wired,* December 13, 2013, wired.com/2013/12/a-calm-look-at-the-most-hyped-concept-in-neuroscience-mirror-neurons/.

Jones, Mary. "History of Meditation." Project-meditation.org, August 5, 2014, project-meditation.org/wim/history_of_meditation.html.

JustAWhisperingGuy. "Things You Should and Should Not Say to ASMRtists," YouTube video, 12:28. December 29, 2012, youtube.com/watch?v=UqdYxt2__24.

Keltner, Dacher. "Hands On Research: The Science of Touch." *Greater Good: The Science of a Meaningful Life,* September 29, 2010, greatergood.berkeley.edu/article/item/hands_on_research.

Kloc, Joe. "The Soothing Sounds of Bob Ross." *Newsweek,* October 1, 2014, newsweek.com/2014/10/10/soothing-sounds-bob-ross-274466.html.

KRBZ in Kansas City. "First ASMR Interview" (MP3 audio file). kcradiogod.com/buzz/ABFMB/asmr0921.mp3.

Lloyd Clarke, Dr. Christopher, MScD. "What Is White Noise? A Clear Explanation At Last!" September 30, 2010, ezinearticles.com/?What-Is-White-Noise?-A-Clear-Explanation-At-Last!&id=5124071.

Lopez, Belinda. "The art and science of whispering." Radiotonic, August 15, 2014, abc.net.au/radionational/programs/radiotonic/the-art-and-science-of-whispering/5672870.

Marshall, Carla. "What It Takes to Make a Living from YouTube's Partner Earnings." ReelSEO.com, October 23, 2013, reelseo.com/youtube-partner-earnings/#partner.

Matt Phil Carver Blog. "ASMR—The sad story of CuteBunny992." February 9, 2014, mattphilcarver.com/blog/asmr-sad-story-cutebunny992/.

Mayo Clinic Staff. "Hypnosis." Mayo Clinic, November 20, 2012, mayoclinic.org/tests-procedures/hypnosis/basics/definition/prc-20019177.

———. "Meditation: A simple, fast way to reduce stress." Mayo Clinic, July 19, 2014, mayoclinic.org/tests-procedures/meditation/in-depth/meditation/art-20045858?pg=1.

Misophonia.com. July 25, 2014.

Mouradian, Sean. "What is the Best Camera or Camcorder for Filming YouTube HD Videos?" Mind Your Money Reviews, February 24, 2014, mymreviews.com/best-camera-for-filming-youtube-videos/.

Myers, Seth, and Katie Gilbert. "The Psychology of Hair Salons and Stylists: Therapy for Free." *Psychology Today,* July 3, 2012, psychologytoday.com/blog/insight-is-2020/201207/the-psychology-hair-salons-stylists-therapy-free.

National Heart, Lung, and Blood Institute. "What Is Sleep Apnea?" July 10, 2012, nhlbi.nih.gov/health/health-topics/topics/sleepapnea/.

National Institute of Neurological Disorders and Stroke. "Narcolepsy." National Institutes of Health, September 11, 2014, ninds.nih.gov/disorders/narcolepsy/detail_narcolepsy.htm.

———. "Restless Legs Syndrome Fact Sheet." National Institutes of Health, July 25, 2014, ninds.nih.gov/disorders/restless_legs/detail_restless_legs.htm.

Nordqvist, Christian. "What is Stress? How to deal with stress." *Medical News Today*, September 5, 2014, medicalnewstoday.com/articles/145855.php.

Novella, Steven. "ASMR." Neurologica Blog, March 12, 2012, theness.com/neurologicablog/index.php/asmr/.

Ofri, Danielle, MD. "Not on the Doctor's Checklist, but Touch Matters." *The New York Times*, August 2, 2010, nytimes.com/2010/08/03/health/03case.html?partner=rss&emc=rss&_r=0.

okaywhatever. "Weird Sensation Feels Good." Steadyhealth.com, December 20, 2010, steadyhealth.com/WEIRD_SENSATION_FEELS_GOOD_t146445.html.

Pearson, Jordan. "Inside the Roleplay Subculture Delivering Tingling 'Braingasms' on YouTube." Motherboard, July 30, 2014, motherboard.vice.com/read/inside-the-roleplay-subculture-delivering-tingling-braingasms-on-youtube.

"Progressive Relaxation Technique." September 12, 2014, stress-relief-tools.com/progressive-relaxation-technique.html.

Psychology World. "Stages of Sleep." July 25, 2014, web.mst.edu/~psyworld/sleep_stages.htm.

Roy, Jessica. "The Internet Gives Me 'Brain Orgasms' and Maybe You Can Get Them Too." *Time*, November 18, 2013, newsfeed.time.com/2013/11/18/the-internet-gives-me-brain-orgasms-and-maybe-you-can-get-them-too/.

Sample, Ian. "Why do we sleep? To clean our brains, say US scientists." *The Guardian*, October 18, 2013, theguardian.com/science/2013/oct/17/sleep-cleans-our-brains-say-scientists.

Shrieves, Linda. "Bob Ross Uses His Brush to Spread Paint and Joy." *Orlando Sentinel*, July 7, 1990, articles.orlandosentinel.com/1990-07-07/lifestyle/9007060122_1_bob-ross-joy-of-painting-pbs?pagewanted=all.

Silady, Alex. "The Economics of ASMR." SmartAsset.com, April 25, 2014, smartasset.com/blog/economics-of/the-economics-of-asmr/.

Stress: Portrait of a Killer. National Geographic documentary, 2008.

Tarakovsky, Margarita, MS. "6 Facts About Transpersonal Psychology." World of Psychology, November 3, 2011, psychcentral.com/blog/archives/2011/11/03/6-facts-about-transpersonal-psychology/.

TheOneLilium. "How to Start Your Own ASMR Channel: 6 Easy Steps! Guidance & Advice," YouTube video, 11:15. August 25, 2014, youtube.com/watch?v=Dw9vbVbWVnA.

Thomas, James P., MD. "Whisper." Voicedoctor.net, September 20, 2014, voicedoctor.net/diagnosis/voice/normal-voice/whisper.

Thompson, Dr. Jeffrey D, DC, BFA. "Methods for Stimulation of Brainwave Function Using Sound." Center for Neuroacoustic Research, 1990, neuroacoustic.com/methods.html.

Transpersonal Hypnotherapy Institute. "Transpersonal Hypnotherapy Described." August 30, 2014, transpersonalhypnotherapy.com/transpersonal-hypnotherapy-described/.

Trex, Ethan. "5 (Happy Little) Things You Didn't Know About Bob Ross." *mental_floss,* November 13, 2009, mentalfloss.com/article/23260/5-happy-little-things-you-didnt-know-about-bob-ross.

University of California—Los Angeles. "Study: Hearing and sight are deeply intertwined." News Medical, December 9, 2011, news-medical.net/news/20111209/Study-Hearing-and-sight-are-deeply-intertwined.aspx.

The Unnamed Feeling. youtube.com/user/UnnamedFeeling13.

———. "ASMR: The Story So Far—A Timeline with History." September 6, 2011, theunnam3df33ling.blogspot.ca/2011/09/asmr-story-so-far-timeline-with-history.html.

Wedmore, James. "Video Camera Reviews: How to Choose the Best Video Camera for YouTube," YouTube video, 11:00. October 2, 2013, youtube.com/watch?v=13MQKzDUUu8.

Weiner, Eli. "Dry-Erase Animation Videos: Why They Work and What You Can Learn." Yes! MediaWorks, February 21, 2013, yesmediaworks.com/blog/bid/113491/Dry-Erase-Animation-Videos-Why-They-Work-and-What-You-Can-Learn You-Can-Learn (site discontinued).

WhisperingLife. "Whisper 1—hello!" YouTube video, 1:46. March 26, 2009, youtube.com/watch?v=IHtgPbfTgKc&list=UUxMEPB9qCXzKViRKW0xmgAw.

———. youtube.com/channel/UCxMEPB9qCXzKViRKW0xmgAw.

Winn, Amanda. "How Certain Sounds Help Us Sleep." Greatist, August 22, 2012, greatist.com/happiness/how-certain-sounds-help-us-sleep.

Wooten, Virgil D., MD. "Natural Sleep Aids." HowStuffWorks, May 16, 2007, health.howstuffworks.com/wellness/natural-medicine/alternative/natural-sleep-aids5.htm.

Young, Julie. "Experiencing ASMR." *Glo Magazine,* September 2013.

Do-It-Yourself Role-Play Props

Looking for some inside tricks to make your role-plays look and sound realistic? Here are a few behind-the-scenes secrets from professional ASMRtists for eight different role-plays! This is hardly an exhaustive list, but it will help get you started. (Remember, not every prop that worked for them will work for you. Each microphone is different, so be sure to test props with your microphone and find the prop that fits your needs.)

Makeup Tutorial Role-Play

This popular role-play is fairly minimal in terms of needed equipment, and chances are you have most of these at your disposal already.

- Makeup bag or case (These not only hold your other props but also can be props themselves if you tap on them, unzip them, or open them carefully.)

- Assorted cosmetics, including foundation, blush, eye shadow, mascara, eyeliner, lipstick, and so on

- Makeup brushes

- Face paint (This is a fun variation on the role-play and can be especially entertaining around Halloween.)

Manicure Role-Play

This is a close relative of the makeup tutorial and salon role-play but contains its own set of tools to make it a relaxing experience. You may already have a lot of these items at your disposal, making it an easy role-play to film. Don't leave anything out!

- Bowl of water

- Fingernail clipper

- Emery board

- Orange stick

- Cuticle trimmer

- Buffer

- Assorted nail polishes

Salon Role-Play

These props are a bit more elaborate and do require some test recordings with your microphone prior to broadcast to ensure you have the sound you hope to re-create. Remember to keep all electronic equipment in a stable location away from the running water.

- Brush, comb, scissors, and other hair-styling equipment

- Plastic sheet to wrap around the "client's" neck

- Running water or spray bottle to wet the "client's" hair

- Towel that can be used to re-create a scalp massage, for a visual aid, or to re-create the hair-washing experience

- Tea bags to re-create a scalp massage (You can hold these next to the microphone to pick up the sound.)

- Sponge and shampoo to recreate a hair-washing experience

- Fake hair or wig to brush and cut (Some ASMRtists use a Barbie head to perform their salon role-plays.)

- Foil sheets and paint brush, if your role-play includes highlights

- Makeup brushes and cosmetics, if your role-play includes a makeup tutorial

Medical Role-Play

Depending on what kind of role-play you are conducting, these props can be pretty elaborate. They can also be very expensive, so where applicable, we have included budget-friendly alternatives.

- Lab coat (You can get these at a costume store or possibly a thrift shop.)
- Latex gloves (These are an amazingly popular auditory trigger.)
- Stethoscope
- Tongue depressors
- Eye chart
- Diagram of whatever body part you are examining
- Bandages
- An otoscope (A small flashlight is usually accepted by the ASMR audience.)
- Wooden mallet (the kind that comes with a child's drum set) to perform reflex tests
- Blood pressure cuff
- Medicinal syringe
- Orange sticks (These are especially effective in ear-cleaning role-plays.)
- Tweezers and a small piece of foam (These are used to simulate ear wax removal.)

Dental Role-Play

This is another role-play that can become very elaborate. While there are some kits you can purchase to make this easier, these are some of the tools you need if you want to start from scratch.

- Fake teeth (These can be improvised by a number of items, including the "gritty side" of ceramic tile or a large lollipop. If there are grooves in it, that's even better!)
- Toothbrush
- Latex gloves
- Dental implements (These can be created with ordinary items, such as a small crochet hook, orange stick, and hard plastic spoon.)

- Dremel drill or electronic toothbrush (This is in the event you are including a filling as part of your role-play.)

- Waterpik water flosser

- Canned air (This is for blowing air on the "client's" teeth.)

Fortune Teller Role-Play

This role-play is always a lot of fun because it is full of interesting, ethereal visuals as well as sounds. It is not the most elaborate role-play, but it is one that needs to be done well in order to be believable.

- Head scarf

- Candles

- Low lighting

- Deck of Tarot cards or regular playing cards to "read" for your client (You will also need some basic explanations of what the cards mean.)

- Gazing ball (This can be improvised by a number of household items, such as a gold fish bowl, a glass bowl, garden orbs, or a glass paperweight.)

- Tea cup and tea leaves to be read

- Star chart (You can add an "astrologer" component to this role-play and include this for zodiac readings.)

Detective Role-Play

Police, detective, and CSI role-plays can be a lot of fun and give you an excuse to dress up and be a little silly with costumes, sounds, and scripts. Some of the props you might need include the following.

- Plastic bags with zip closures

- Large tweezers

- Magnifying glass

- Paper bag (This is for larger pieces of "evidence.")

- Spray bottle (You use this to simulate Luminol, which in police terms picks up traces of blood.)

- Paintbrush or electromagnetic duster

- White powder (This is to dust for fingerprints.)

Interior Designer Role-Play

This role-play is fun because it's usually not too difficult to find the props you need to make this work, and the sounds you make tapping and scratching the different surfaces will seem incredible to your audience. The key to this role-play is texture and variety.

- Carpet samples

- Paint chips

- Countertop samples

- Ceramic, glass, or natural stone tiles (If possible, get a wide variety of varying textures to create a sonic symphony for your viewer.)

- Fabric swatches (Again, variety is key.)

- Drapery accessories, such as tassels, beads, finials, and hooks

- Lampshades, especially pleated ones

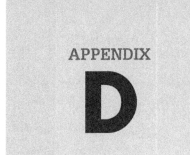

APPENDIX

D

Sample Script for ASMR Role-Play

Are you ready to create your own ASMR content but hate the thought of researching and writing that first script? If so, this sample script will help you film one of the most popular ASMR role-plays: a 15-minute cranial nerve examination. Remember that this is only a sample, and something you can add to or subtract from as necessary, or customize as you see fit.

Props:

- Ball-point pen (preferably one that clicks)

- Clipboard and paper (can be a copy of this script to help keep your video on track)

- Computer and keyboard or laptop

- Small flashlight (a penlight works best)

- Color chart (can be one you print or one you make)

- 2 small plastic or glass containers with screw-on lids

- 2 spray bottles filled with water (can be different colors so that your viewer can distinguish them)

- Cotton swab

- Orange stick

[The scene opens with you, the ASMRTIST, typing on your keyboard with your attention fixed on the computer screen. After a brief moment, take note of the VIEWER with a slight double-take before speaking.]

ASMRTIST

Oh, hello, welcome to our clinic. What can I do for you today?

[Gaze gently at the screen and pause long enough for the VIEWER to say she has come for a cranial nerve examination. Nod.]

ASMRTIST

A cranial nerve exam? Of course. Do you have an appointment?

[Pause long enough for the VIEWER to confirm that she has an appointment for two o'clock.]

ASMRTIST

Two o'clock? Let me look that up for you.

[Turn your attention back to the computer screen in order to verify the VIEWER'S appointment.]

Your name?

[Pause before glancing back at the camera.]

Can I get you to spell that for me?

[Pause for a moment before nodding and typing the VIEWER'S name. (If you are unsure of what name to type, use your own.)]

Date of birth?

Pause.

And is this your first visit to the clinic, or is this a follow-up appointment?

[Pause long enough to "hear" the VIEWER say that this is a follow-up visit and then tap any key as if checking a box.]

Have there been any changes to your condition since your last visit?

[Pause and tap a key again.]

And are you allergic to any medication?

[Pause and tap a key again.]

ASMRTIST

[Turn your attention back to the camera and smile gently.]

Okay, let's begin. My name is *(insert personal name or screen name)* and I will be administering your cranial nerve examination today. As you know, the cranial nerve exam is part of an overall neurological examination and one that is designed to identify problems in the cranial nerves.

The examination is comprised of 12 tests with a few subtests contained within. When I complete this series of tests, I will be able to tell you if I have any concerns. Do you have any questions before I begin?

[Pause long enough for the VIEWER to ask if it will hurt.]

ASMRTIST

[Shake your head.]

No, it will not hurt, and you should not feel any pain or discomfort. It will be just like last time, okay?

[Pause for assent.]

ASMRTIST

Great, let's begin. The first thing I am going to test is your olfactory nerve, which is your sense of smell. This will help me identify any problems in the nasal passages that could indicate a possible nerve lesion or a deviated septum.

I am going to ask you to close your right nostril while I place a sample scent under the left one for identification purposes.

[Begin preparing a sample off-camera by deliberately unscrewing the lid off of one of the jars and gently dragging the lid across the mouth or rim of the container. You may also gently tap on its side, if you wish, for an extra tingle trigger. Hold the jar out toward the camera.]

ASMRTIST

Okay, breathe in … can you tell me what it is?

[Gaze patiently and wait long enough for the VIEWER to say "cinnamon."]

Um-hmmm, cinnamon is correct. Now let's try this one. It's a little different because it is in a spray bottle.

[Hold the spray bottle up and gently shake it so the VIEWER can hear the liquid. Off-camera, squeeze the trigger on the mister so the VIEWER can hear it. You can also tap it on the side as you did with the jar for an extra tingle trigger.]

Breathe in … can you identify the smell?

[Pause for a minute so the VIEWER can tell you it is "pine."]

Very good. That is correct. Now let's switch sides. Cover up your left nostril so I can test the right one.

[Demonstrate what it is the VIEWER is supposed to do, smile gently, and then prepare the third sample in the same way you did the first with the lidded jar.]

Okay, breathe in again … very good … can you tell me what you smell?

[Pause long enough for the VIEWER to identify "cloves."]

Um-hmm, cloves is correct. Now I have one more for you ….

[Take the second spray bottle and prepare it the same way you did the first one, shaking the bottle so the VIEWER can hear it. Then squeeze the trigger off-camera.]

And … breathe in ….

[Pause.]

You need it one more time?

[Nod and mist the spray bottle once again.]

Can you tell me what you smell?

[Pause long enough for the VIEWER to identify "lemon."]

Lemon, yes … very good.

[Click open your pen and make four check marks on your clipboard.]

ASMRTIST

For our next test, I will evaluate your optic nerve. This will help us identify any issues with your visual acuity and check for optic neuritis. Do you wear glasses or contacts?

[Pause long enough for the VIEWER to say "no."]

Okay, let's continue. What I am going to do is ask you to cover your right eye and keep your left eye focused on the tip of my nose.

[Cover your own eye to demonstrate this and tap the tip of your nose for effect.]

I am going to test your peripheral vision by wiggling my finger off to the side. I want you to tell me when you see it, okay?

[Randomly test the four quadrants of the VIEWER'S peripheral vision by wiggling your finger. Pause after every wiggle as if the VIEWER has spotted it and identified the movement. Offer an "um-hmm" after every wiggle. Do this 4 or 5 times.]

Okay, now let's test the other side. Go ahead and uncover your right eye and cover your left. Remember to keep your right eye on the tip of my nose.

[Repeat the peripheral vision test on the other side using the same movements as before. Do this 4 or 5 times.]

Very good … let me make a few notes ….

[Pick up the clipboard and click the pen to jot some notes.]

ASMRTIST

Now I am going to show you some colors on this chart, and I want you to tell me if you can identify them.

[Hold up the color chart, or if mounted on a wall, use your pen to indicate which color you want identified. Plan to ask about 6 or 7 colors, offering an "um-hmm" after every correct response.]

Very good. Now I need to perform a fundoscopy, in which I will test how your pupils react to bright light. I need you to cover your right eye again while I shine this light into your left ….

[Hold up small flashlight for the VIEWER to see.]

No, you do not have to look at my nose this time. Just stare straight ahead … very good ….

[Turn on the flashlight and aim it directly at the camera while placing your hand above as if to simulate having your hand on the VIEWER'S head.]

ASMRTIST

All right, now we'll look at the other eye. If I could have you open your right eye and cover your left … that's it. Thank you.

[Aim the flashlight directly at the camera again and repeat placing your hand above the camera as if to have your hand on the patient's head.]

Okay. Now you can open up both eyes. And if I could get you to follow the light with both eyes for me ….

[Slowly swing the flashlight back and forth.]

Okay, very good, you can relax now.

[Pick up the pen and clipboard to make a few notes.]

ASMRTIST

Okay, now I am just going to inspect your eyes for any abnormalities and asymmetry, so let me take a look here ….

[Place your hand above the camera or at the side to simulate spreading the VIEWER'S eye open for observation. Gaze gently at the camera, making sure to shift your own eyes as though you are actually looking into the VIEWER'S eyes. Repeat this test on each side.]

Okay, now I am going to move my finger in a pattern in front of you and I am going to ask you to follow it with just your eyes—not your head; just your eyes.

[Make an "H" shape with your fingers a few times and then smile gently when the VIEWER has successfully finished the test.]

And now I am going to bring my fingers close to your nose …

[Demonstrate.]

… and away ….

[Demonstrate.]

Okay, very good.

[Pick up the pen and make some more notes on the clipboard.]

ASMRTIST

This next test will evaluate your trigeminal nerve. This is known as the light-touch test, and I will start by taking this cotton swab …

[Hold up the cotton swab so the VIEWER can see it.]

… and moving it across your jawline. Then I will move on to your cheek, your forehead, and then test your corneal reflex.

[Start by moving the cotton swab just below the camera to simulate testing the jawline. When you are finished, move on to the cheek, announcing each facial feature as it is tested. (Some ASMRTISTS augment this test by lightly dragging the cotton swab across the microphone.)]

Now I'm going to do this once again, but this time with this orange stick ….

[Hold up the orange stick for the VIEWER to see.]

Yes, I know it has a point, but it will not hurt ….

[Repeat the test as before.]

Very good. Now I will test the corneal reflex on your left eye using this cotton swab …. Go ahead and close your right eye for me.

[Bring the cotton swab toward the camera, but do not touch it. (In a real corneal reflex test, the VIEWER would automatically blink as the object comes closer to her eye.)]

And now the other side. Close your left eye for me ….

[Repeat the movement.]

Very good.

[Pick up the pen and check off more imaginary boxes on the clipboard paper. Nod as you make notes.]

ASMRTIST

Oh yes, you are doing fine. See, I told you there was nothing to worry about. This is the easiest test you will ever take.

[Smile. Put down the clipboard and turn your attention back to the VIEWER.]

What I need you to do now is clench your teeth together so I can feel your muscles for any irregularities.

[Feel along the VIEWER'S jawline and forehead by moving your hands just below and just above the camera lens.]

Now I am going to put my hand under your chin, and I want you to try and open your mouth against the resistance.

[Place your hand directly under the camera lens; pause and smile.]

Very good. Now I will inspect your facial nerves, which will help me note any facial asymmetry and involuntary movements that could indicate the possibility of Bell's palsy or Ramsay Hunt syndrome. Can I get you to raise your eyebrows for me?

[Demonstrate this action and pause so the VIEWER can do it as well. Pause briefly.]

Very good. Can you frown for me?

[Again, demonstrate this action so the VIEWER can see what you mean. Pause briefly.]

And … can you puff out your cheeks for me?

[Demonstrate this action so the VIEWER can see it; pause and smile.]

And now if I could see your teeth?

[Demonstrate and pause.]

Do it again, please?

[Pause.]

Okay, very good.

[Pick up the pen and make notes on the clipboard.]

ASMRTIST

Now I am going to test your hearing by whispering a series of numbers in your ears and having you repeat them to me. I will start on your right side ….

[Lean toward the right side of the camera from the VIEWER's perspective (which will be on your left side). You can also administer this test by standing up and moving behind the camera so the VIEWER does not know which ear you will be testing. (This is especially effective if you are using a binaural microphone or other specialized equipment.) Whisper five numbers between 1 and 50 randomly.]

And now the other side.

[Repeat the test on the other ear if you are not administering the test randomly in order to achieve anticipatory tingles. Make notes on the clipboard when finished.]

ASMRTIST

Very good. Now I need to have a look inside your mouth. This will help me assess your glossopharyngeal and vagus nerves …. What's the matter …? Oh, you didn't brush your teeth? Don't worry about it. You aren't the first … you won't be the last. Open up your mouth please so that I can have a look ….

[Turn on the flashlight again and shine it directly under the camera but just enough to where the VIEWER can see a hint of the light.]

Um-hmm, that looks really good. Now stick out your tongue and move it from side to side ….

[Demonstrate and pause.]

Very good.

[Make more notes on the clipboard.]

ASMRTIST

Now the last thing I want to do is test the muscles in your neck and shoulder area. I am just going to place my hands on your shoulders in order to create some resistance ….

[Reach out toward the camera as if to place your hands on the VIEWER'S shoulders.]

Now can you try and shrug your shoulders?

[Pause and smile.]

Very good, and if I pull your shoulders forward, can you try and bring them back …?

[Pause.]

Very good. Now I am just going to put my hands on either side of your face ….

[Place your hands on either side of the camera lens.]

And I want you to try and move your head to the right ….

[Pause.]

Now to the left ….

[Pause.]

Okay, great.

ASMRTIST

[Gather the clipboard one more time and make final notes on the VIEWER'S chart. These notes can be a bit more extensive than previous ones.]

Okay, so that concludes your cranial nerve examination. Do you have any questions?

[Pause long enough for the VIEWER to ask how long it will take to get the results.]

You will get your official results within a few days, but I can assure you that I did not see any abnormalities during the assessment. You really have nothing to worry about.

[Pause.]

No, I don't see any reason that you would need to come back … just stay healthy, let me know if you have any problems, and in the meantime, have a great night.

[Smile.]

The End

The Top 100 ASMRtists

ASMRtist Paul Artwork collected this list for a research presentation that was published on his YouTube channel on June 20, 2014. The rankings are based on channel views rather than subscribers or particular videos. While they do change from time to time based on "hits," this will give you a sense of the top ASMRtists you can explore on YouTube.

1. **GentleWhispering** (youtube.com/user/GentleWhispering/featured): A few popular uploads of this ASMRtist are a 3D sounds video, a 3D haircut role-play, and a binaural spa role-play.

2. **Heather Feather** (youtube.com/user/HeatherFeatherASMR): Heather has done videos such as a binaural cranial nerve examination; an ASMR trigger video; and a binaural sounds panning video for sleep, tingles, and relaxation.

3. **MassageASMR** (youtube.com/user/MassageASMR): At her channel, you can find videos that include a relaxing role-play session with an ASMRtist, a relaxing back massage, and a head and face massage session.

4. **TheWaterwhispers** (youtube.com/user/TheWaterwhispers): Some of the most popular videos she has made are an ASMR trigger video, a soft-spoken binaural ear examination, and a long whisper session for sleep and relaxation.

5. **ASMRrequests** (youtube.com/user/ASMRrequests): A sci-fi role-play, a binaural face massage role-play, and a face brushing video with whispering and soft speaking are just a few of the popular videos found on this channel.

6. **Ephemeral Rift** (youtube.com/user/EphemeralRift): At this ASMRtist's channel, you can find videos such as a woodland nature sounds video, a candy man role-play, and an ASMR test subject role-play.

7. **VeniVidiVulpes** (youtube.com/user/VeniVidiVulpes): A few of the most popular role-plays she has created are a virtual spa haircut role-play, a men's haircut and razor shave role-play, and a relaxing makeover with soft speaking and whispering.

8. **TheOneLilium** (youtube.com/user/TheOneLilium): At her channel, you can find a close-up 3D microphone test video, a lucid dreaming experiment, a 3D sounds and close-up ASMR trigger video, and many others.

9. **asmrmassage** (youtube.com/user/asmrmassage): A hair play head massage session, a back tickle massage video, and an Indian head massage role-play are just a few of the most viewed videos on this ASMRtist's channel.

10. **Pigsbum53 ASMR** (youtube.com/user/pigsbum53): Some of her most popular videos are an ASMR healing therapy role-play, a Korean scalp scratching and ear cleaning role-play, and a spa facial role-play.

11. **amalzd** (youtube.com/user/amalzd): At this channel, you can watch videos such as a spa role-play, an ASMR bra-fitting role-play, and a librarian role-play.

12. **WhisperCrystal** (youtube.com/user/WhisperCrystal): Some of the most popular videos at this ASMRtist's channel are a soft-spoken paradise island massage role-play, a Turkish bath massage role-play, and a peaceful whisper session for sleep and relaxation.

13. **VisualSounds1** (youtube.com/user/VisualSounds1): A few of her most well-known videos include a ASMR visual sounds trigger session, a nail tapping video, and a brushing on canvas video.

14. **WhispersUnicorn** (youtube.com/user/WhispersUnicorn): A soft-spoken cosmetology role-play, a soft-spoken reading video, and a haircut role-play are just a few options you can check out on this channel.

15. **softlygaloshes** (youtube.com/user/softlygaloshes): The most popular videos you can explore from this ASMRtist are a binaural ear-to-ear whisperfest, a binaural trigger video, and an unintelligible whispering video.

16. **Olivia's Kissper ASMR** (youtube.com/user/OliviaKissperASMR): Some of her most popular videos are a binaural hair play, a binaural ASMR trigger video, and an Indian head and scalp massage session.

17. **SOUNDsculptures** (youtube.com/user/SOUNDsculptures): At this channel, you can find a 3D sounds-only scalp massage and hair washing session, a virtual barber shop role-play, a water marble sounds video, and more.

18. **QueenOfSerene** (youtube.com/user/QueenOfSerene): A relaxing facial and scalp massage role-play, a gentleman's suit fitting role-play, and an ASMR tapping and scratching video are some of the options you can find at this channel.

19. **thatASMRchick** (youtube.com/user/thatASMRchick): A few of her most popular videos are a binaural microphone touching video, a scalp massage and ear cleaning role-play, and a inaudible whisper session.

20. Hailey WhisperingRose (youtube.com/user/Hlvillaire): Some of this ASMRtist's best-known videos are a 3D scalp massage role-play, a cuddle time role-play, and a haircut role-play.

21. Fairy Char ASMR (youtube.com/user/feirychaRstaRs): Her channel has a 3D scalp massage with ear-to-ear whispering, an ASMR hair brushing video, an ear cleaning role-play, and more.

22. Tony Bomboni (ASMRer) (youtube.com/user/Asmrer): At this ASMRtist's channel, you can find videos such as a binaural ear and head exam role-play, a faerie role-play, and a binaural makeover role-play.

23. Sweetseductiveasmr (youtube.com/user/Sweetseductiveasmr): A few videos this ASMRtist is well known for are a crinkly bag session; a face massage video; and a relaxing tapping, scratching, and tracing video for sleep and relaxation.

24. RelaxingASMR (youtube.com/user/RelaxingASMR): A vintage writing sounds video, a "fall write to sleep" writing session, and a pocket knife sharpening ASMR whisper video are just a selection of ASMR content you can find here.

25. Asmraurette (channel has been deactivated): While Asmraurette has unfortunately deactivated her channel, she was known for her guided visual relaxation, trigger words, and gender-neutral make-up role-play videos.

26. ASMRGRAINS (youtube.com/user/WhisperMister1): A few of his most popular videos are a haircut/shave role-play for men, a cranial nerve examination role-play, and a male grooming session.

27. SavannahsVoice (youtube.com/user/SavannahsVoice): At this channel, you can check out videos such as a soft-spoken hypnosis session for sleep and relaxation, a whisper video, and a present wrapping video.

28. CalmingEscape (youtube.com/user/CalmingEscape): The most watched uploads to this channel are a haircut/styling role-play, a hypnotist role-play, and a scalp check role-play.

29. ASMRmania (youtube.com/user/ASMRmania): Some of her most popular video are a Russian doctor role-play, a medical exam role-play and a tourist agency role-play.

30. ThePeacefulWhisper (youtube.com/user/ThePeacefulWhisper): A few of her most popular videos are a massage therapist role-play, a beauty routine whisper video and an antique dealer role-play.

31. asmrnovaster (youtube.com/user/asmrnovastar): A virtual massage role-play, a cranial nerve examination, and an ear-to-ear whisper video for sleep induction are among the videos offered on this channel.

32. JustAWhisperingGuy (youtube.com/user/JustAWhisperingGuy): At this channel, you can find videos such as a binaural ear touching session for sleep and relaxation, a binaural ear examination role-play, and a two-hour-long ASMR video.

33. TheUKASMR (youtube.com/user/TheUKASMR): A barber shop role-play, a hairdresser role-play with hair washing sounds, and a dreamy spa role-play are just a few videos you can find through this ASMRtist.

34. whispersweetie (youtube.com/user/whispersweetie): Some of her most popular videos are a hand relaxation video, a body and scalp massage role-play, and a relaxing sounds video.

35. VioletsVoice (youtube.com/user/VioletsVoice): This channel offers uploads such as a binaural ear-to-ear whispering session, a binaural studio sounds video, and a loving partner affirmation role-play.

36. kiwiwhispers ASMR (youtube.com/user/kiwiwhispers): You can find a binaural 3D relaxing piano sounds music video, a panning whisper video, and a doctor's appointment role-play with audio only among other videos at this ASMRtist's channel.

37. AppreciateASMR (youtube.com/user/AppreciateASMR): A relaxing haircut role-play, a close-up guided journey of the senses, and a 3D relaxing makeover role-play are just a few options you can check out at this channel.

38. DonnaASMR (youtube.com/user/DonnaASMR): A few of this ASMRtist's most popular videos include a microphone touching, scratching, and brushing video; a Kinder surprise egg unwrapping video; and a show-and-tell video about games.

39. softsoundwhispers (youtube.com/user/softsoundwhispers): At this channel, you can find videos such as a face brushing session, a haircut role-play, and a hair brushing video.

40. Asmr Vids (youtube.com/user/asmrVids): Some of his most well-known videos are a sculpting toy video, a Zen garden video, and a cake baking video.

41. Air Light (youtube.com/user/AirLightASMR): A binaural mouth sounds and ear-to-ear whispering video, a multilayers deep binaural ASMR session, and a binaural ASMR head massage video with shampooing sounds can be found at this channel.

42. ASMRvelous (youtube.com/user/ASMRvelous): This ASMRtist's most well-known uploads are a soft-spoken guided sleep relaxation video, a touching hands and neck whisper video, and a soft-spoken therapist role-play.

43. SilentCitadel (youtube.com/user/SilentCitadel): This channel includes videos such as a relaxing hand massage video, a tarot card reading session, and a tapping and scratching of different objects video.

44. Th3HazySea (youtube.com/user/Th3HazySea): Some of her most popular videos are a doctor check-up role-play, a teacher role-play, and a cranial nerve examination role-play.

45. Sachi_asmr (youtube.com/user/sckhre): At this channel, you can find a personal role-play with up close sounds, a trigger video with different sounds, a show-and-tell video about candy, and more.

46. adreambeam (youtube.com/user/adreambeam): A relaxing makeup artist role-play, an eye doctor exam, and a sales girl role-play are just a few popular options at this channel.

47. Amandaine LeloupAsmr (channel no longer active): While her channel is sadly not active anymore, she was known for ASMR-friendly content in French.

48. Christen Noel (youtube.com/user/ChristenNoelASMR): This ASMRtist is known for videos like a haircut role-play, a 20 ASMR trigger video, and a binaural whisper video that includes touching and brushing a microphone.

49. DianaDew Asmr (youtube.com/user/DianaDewAsmr): At this channel, you can explore videos such as an ear-to-ear wet mouth sounds video, an intense and breathy ear-to-ear session, and a spa role-play with ear cleaning.

50. fastASMR (youtube.com/user/fastASMR): Some of her most popular videos are a fast tapping video session, an ear-to-ear video with slow hand movements, and a binaural ear cleaning role-play.

51. Mitzy Whispers (youtube.com/user/mitzypieful): This channel offers videos such as a hair dye role-play, a relaxing scalp massage session, and a Reiki role-play.

52. whisperflower (youtube.com/user/whisperflower): A studying whisper video, a clipping coupons video, and a rambling in Russian video are all offered at this ASMRtist's channel.

53. softlywhispered (youtube.com/user/softlywhispered): You can check out videos such as an ear examination role-play, a doctor's check-up role-play, and a relaxing eye examination role-play here.

54. ASMRlove (youtube.com/user/ASMRlove): This ASMRtist is known for videos like a salon and haircut role-play, a facial massage role-play, and a scratching and tapping on various objects video.

55. ASMR Angel (youtube.com/user/TheASMRAngel): A few of this ASMRtist's most popular videos are a cranial nerve examination role-play, a close-up ear-to-ear inaudible whisper video, and a binaural ear examination role-play.

56. NeonIndieGirl (youtube.com/user/NeonIndieGirl): At this channel, you can find a lip smacking and whispering video, a head massage with hair brushing video, and a cranial nerve examination role-play.

57. WhispersRedASMR (youtube.com/user/WhispersRedASMR): A childhood memories ASMR trigger video, a medical exam role-play, and a deep ear cleaning role-play are some of the videos available at this channel.

58. MissMeridianASMR (youtube.com/user/MissMeridianASMR): This channel includes videos such as a whispered sleep guide that includes kissing and lip smacking sounds, a trigger sounds video, and a scalp scratching and shoulder massage video.

59. Brittany ASMR (youtube.com/user/BrittanyASMR): Some of the most popular videos from this ASMRtist are an unintelligible and inaudible ear-to-ear whisper session, a "let me help you sleep" video, and a video-game collection show-and-tell.

60. quietexperiment (youtube.com/user/quietexperiment): At this channel, you can check out uploads like a binaural whisper and sounds session, an animated binaural sounds video, and a tapping and scratching on a go-board and stones video.

61. Deep Ocean of Sounds (youtube.com/user/DeepOceanOfsounds): A few of the well-known videos on this channel are a virtual hairdresser/barber shop sounds-only video, a binaural scratching your head sounds video, and a brushing and tapping sound session.

62. AuroraWhispers (youtube.com/user/AuroraWhispers): A sounds-only full-body massage spa experience role-play, a relaxing soft-spoken shiatsu role-play, and a facial massage role-play that includes music are some options you can find on this channel.

63. MaleSoothe (youtube.com/user/MaleSoothe): Some of his most accessed videos are a make-over role-play, a sleep hypnosis and relaxation video, and a doctor visit role-play.

64. Lauren Ostrowski Fenton (youtube.com/user/laurenlouisefenton): This ASMRtist has created videos such as an instruction video on how to meditate for beginners, a makeup role-play, and a preparation for deeper sleep session.

65. TheLyricalWhispers (youtube.com/user/TheLyricalWhispers): At this channel, you can find videos such as a cranial nerve examination, a haircut role-play, and an eye examination role-play.

66. LauraLemureX ASMR (youtube.com/user/LauraLemureX): A trigger word assortment video, a semi-inaudible ear-to-ear whisper video, and a scalp massage role-play are just a few videos available on this channel.

67. tahteebayy (youtube.com/user/tahteebayy): A few of this ASMRtist's most popular videos are an eating sounds video, a inaudible mouth noises video, and a chewing gum whisper video.

68. ardra neala (youtube.com/user/ardraneala): You can explore videos like a binaural psionic initiation role-play, a sound assortment video, and a mystic healer role-play through this ASMRtist's channel.

69. whisperslily (youtube.com/user/whisperslily): This ASMRtist is known for videos such as a soft-spoken cranial nerve examination role-play, a whispered spa role-play, and a makeover role-play.

70. asmrkitten (youtube.com/user/asmrkitten): Some of the more popular options through this ASMRtist are a "let me ASMR you" session, a cranial nerve examination, and a binaural tattoo consultation role-play.

71. Urara1966 ASMR (youtube.com/user/urara1966): A Japanese ear picking video, a binaural sounds video, and a 3D sounds video are a few of the uploads you can find at this ASMRtist's channel.

72. xOMelissOx (ASMR material has been deleted): At this channel, you can explore videos such as a tapping and scratching video with long nails, a book scratching video, and a tapping and scratching on random objects video.

73. TrixiWhispers ASMR (youtube.com/user/TrixiWhispers): A few of her most viewed videos are a head massage demonstration session, a smoothing crinkled paper sounds video, and a crinkly and sticky fingers sounds video.

74. WhisperingLife (youtube.com/user/WhisperingLife): This ASMRtist is known for videos such as a whisper video, a reading *Harry Potter* video, and a doodling with whispering video.

75. UnicornsWhisper (youtube.com/user/UnicornsWhisper): A head spa role-play, a guided deep sleep relaxation video, and a spa role-play for men in Russian highlight this ASMRtist's channel.

76. Relaxingsounds92 (youtube.com/user/Relaxingsounds92): At this channel, you can check out offerings such as a tapping and scratching video; a nail tapping on one surface session; and a crinkly plastic, paper, and sticky finger sounds video.

77. WhisperingHands4You (youtube.com/user/WhisperingHands4You): Some of this ASMRtist's most popular videos are a makeup role-play, a clothing store role-play, and a mini spa role-play.

78. ASMRsoundandnoises (youtube.com/user/ASMRsoundandnoises): This ASMRtist has uploads such as a haircut and hand massage role-play, an eye exam role-play, and a makeover role-play.

79. albinwhisperland (youtube.com/user/albinwhisperland): You can explore videos such as a gentle hair play video, a makeup collection show-and-tell video, and a soft-spoken comic book recommendations role-play through this channel.

80. Makoto.ASMR (youtube.com/user/makoto7102): An ear cleaning and ear picking video, a makeup role-play, and a 3D ear massage role-play are some of the video offerings through this ASMRtist.

81. amsrdidibandy (youtube.com/user/didibandy): A few of her most popular videos are a real-life back massage role-play, a doctor role-play, and a cranial nerve examination role-play.

82. Lilliwhispers (youtube.com/user/Lilliwhispers): At this channel, you can find videos like a makeup artist role-play, a show-and-tell with gum chewing sounds video, and a flight attendant role-play.

83. MissBunnyWhispers (youtube.com/user/MissBunnyWhispers): Some highlights of this ASMRtist's channel are a cranial nerve examination role-play, a men's head massage session, and an ASMR trigger video without talking.

84. Nicolasmrelaxation (youtube.com/user/Nicolasmrelaxation): This channel provides videos such as a haircut role-play, a French whisper video, and a French nerve examination role-play.

85. SoftAnnaPL (youtube.com/user/SoftAnnaPL): A Polish whisper video with inaudible whispering and microphone blowing, a virtual dentist role-play in Polish, and an ear-to-ear Polish whisper video with mouth sounds are some of the most viewed videos from this ASMRtist.

86. Hermetic Kitten (youtube.com/user/hermetickitten): You can explore a Spanish spoken multilayered ear-to-ear video, a blue yeti microphone test video, a binaural words video, and more through this channel.

87. RandomSarahGrace (youtube.com/user/randomsarahgrace): A few of her well-known videos are a page-turning trigger video, a glamour nail tapping video, and a brushing the camera lens session.

88. Ariel ASMR (youtube.com/user/letmebeyourefantasy): At this channel, you can check out videos such as a playing with hair and makeup on a Barbie head video, a Reiki healing session, and a mesmerizing visual sounds compilation.

89. 17MissCoco (youtube.com/user/17MissCoco): A follow the pen session in German, a beauty salon role-play in German, and a cranial nerve examination in German highlight the options this ASMRtist offers.

90. Sirène Bio (youtube.com/user/elisaboelle): Some of her most popular videos are a French whisper show-and-tell video, a guided relaxation session in French, and a playing with dice video.

91. ASMR HQ (youtube.com/user/asmrhq): This channel offers uploads such as a kinetic sand demonstration, a binaural sounds video, and a magic milk color experiment.

92. ASMR Destiny (youtube.com/user/asmrdestiny): This ASMRtist's channel has videos including a binaural ear cupping video, an ear cleaning video, and an inaudible whisper video.

93. JubileeWhispers (youtube.com/user/JubileeWhispers): At this channel, you can explore videos like a 3D ear-to-ear whisper video, a binaural cranial nerve examination, and a relaxing spa role-play.

94. accidentallygraceful (youtube.com/user/accidentallygraceful): This ASMRtist is known for videos such as a natural bath salt recipe tutorial, a perfect spa bath video, and a scalp massage session.

95. ASMR By Design (youtube.com/user/ASMRByDesign): Some of the more popular options on this channel are a massage video with sounds and unintelligible whispering, a full-body relaxation session, and a Lego kit building video.

96. Paul Artwork (youtube.com/user/PaulSimardPsy): At this channel, you can find videos such as a haircut role-play, an eye exam and pure light trigger video, and a sketching video with soft brushing.

97. theASMRnerd (youtube.com/user/theASMRnerd): A few of his most popular videos are a sorting Pokémon cards video, a gaming whisper video, and an ASMR whisper video.

98. MissGumbyASMR (youtube.com/user/MissGumbyASMR): A Spanish hypnosis session for sleep, a cranial nerve examination role-play, and a candy sounds video are just a few examples of what's offered through this ASMRtist.

99. ASMR Sounds by Sophie / Xcentricity Body Painting (youtube.com/user/chalicemagic): This channel includes a whispered doodling video, a Celtic knot-work drawing video, and a body art with henna video.

100. WillowsWhisper (youtube.com/user/EllyBellyBoo123): Some highlights of this ASMRtist's channel are a cranial nerve examination, a haircut role-play, and an eye examination video.

Index

W-X-Y-Z

Printed in Great Britain
by Amazon

42521782R00152